THE CLINICAL LABORATORY MANUAL SERIES:

Hematology

Other Delmar titles in this Clinical Laboratory Manual Series include:

Dean/Whitlock: The Clinical Laboratory Manual Series: Clinical Chemistry
Flynn/Whitlock: The Clinical Laboratory Manual Series: Urinalysis
Hoeltke: The Clinical Laboratory Manual Series: Phlebotomy
Marshall: The Clinical Laboratory Manual Series: Microbiology
Smith: The Clinical Laboratory Manual Series: Immunology
Whitlock: The Clinical Laboratory Manual Series: Immunohematology

Also available from Delmar Publishers:

Davis: Phlebotomy: A Client-Based Approach
Fong/Lakomia: Microbiology for Health Careers, 5E
Hoeltke: The Complete Textbook of Phlebotomy
Marshall: Fundamental Skills for the Clinical Laboratory Professional
Walters: Basic Medical Laboratory Techniques, 3E

THE CLINICAL LABORATORY MANUAL SERIES:

Hematology

Allan Paul Russell, EdD, RMT (ISCLT)

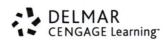

DELMAR
CENGAGE Learning

Australia • Brazil • Japan • Korea • Mexico • Singapore • Spain • United Kingdom • United States

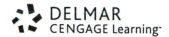
DELMAR
CENGAGE Learning™

The Clinical Laboratory Manual Series:
Hematology
Allan Paul Russell

Publisher: Susan Simpfenderfer

Acquisitions Editor: Marion Waldman

Project Editor: William Trudell

Art and Design Coordinator: Rich Killar

Production Coordinator: John Mickelbank

Editorial Assistant: Sarah Holle

Marketing Manager: Darryl L. Caron

Cover Design: Joanne Beckmann Design

For product information and technology assistance, contact us at
Cengage Learning Customer & Sales Support, 1-800-354-9706

For permission to use material from this text or product,
submit all requests online at **cengage.com/permissions**
Further permissions questions can be emailed to
permissionrequest@cengage.com

Library of Congress Control Number: 96-18847

ISBN-13: 978-0-8273-6373-1

ISBN-10: 0-8273-6373-7

Delmar
Executive Woods
5 Maxwell Drive
Clifton Park, NY 12065
USA

Cengage Learning is a leading provider of customized learning solutions with office locations around the globe, including Singapore, the United Kingdom, Australia, Mexico, Brazil, and Japan. Locate your local office at:
international.cengage.com/region

Cengage Learning products are represented in Canada by Nelson Education, Ltd.

For your lifelong learning solutions, visit **delmar.cengage.com**

Visit our corporate website at **www.cengage.com**

Notice to the Reader
Publisher does not warrant or guarantee any of the products described herein or perform any independent analysis in connection with any of the product information contained herein. Publisher does not assume, and expressly disclaims, any obligation to obtain and include information other than that provided to it by the manufacturer. The reader is expressly warned to consider and adopt all safety precautions that might be indicated by the activities described herein and to avoid all potential hazards. By following the instructions contained herein, the reader willingly assumes all risks in connection with such instructions. The publisher makes no representations or warranties of any kind, including but not limited to, the warranties of fitness for particular purpose or merchantability, nor are any such representations implied with respect to the material set forth herein, and the publisher takes no responsibility with respect to such material. The publisher shall not be liable for any special, consequential, or exemplary damages resulting, in whole or part, from the readers' use of, or reliance upon, this material.

Printed in the United States of America
11 12 13 14 15   14 13 12 11 10
ED144

Thanks to my wife, Shirley,
our children, Bonnie, Lora, and Allan, Jr.,
and my mother, Rita,
for their love and support

CONTENTS

■ Contents

LIST OF LABORATORY EXERCISES

PREFACE

This hematology manual was developed to meet the need for laboratory experience for students involved in the clinical laboratory sciences. It utilizes eighty-nine laboratory exercises to give the student a hands-on approach to the field. The student can actively participate in each exercise to gain the skills needed to understand the basic principles of hematology.

The exercises are set up as laboratory procedures with a purpose, equipment needed, and a step-by-step procedure to arrive at the result. Students are encouraged to seek information in reference textbooks to add to the experience with this manual.

I would like to acknowledge the help of my colleagues who contributed to the completion of this manual: Christine Kisiel, Linda LaRoche, and Renee Herold, who helped locate information for me. The reviewers helped me to chart a course. Special thanks go to Jackie Marshall for her assistance in editing this manual.

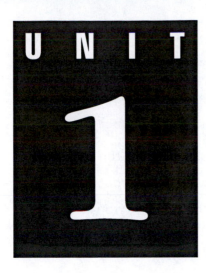

UNIT 1

Introduction to Hematology in the Clinical Laboratory

LEARNING OBJECTIVES

Having completed this unit, it is the responsibility of the student to know the following:

- Define the term hematology.

- List the components of blood.

- Discuss safety issues in the hematology laboratory.

- Explain Universal Precautions.

- List techniques to operate electrical equipment safely in the laboratory.

- Explain how to operate a microscope.

- Describe blood cell organelles.

GLOSSARY

absorbance amount of detectable light absorbed into a sample.

chromatin combination of DNA and histones forming the chromosomes.

cytoplasm water and chemicals found within the plasma membrane.

endoplasmic reticulum channels found within the cellular cytoplasm.

filaments strands of visible nuclear material between larger amounts of nuclear material.

formed elements another name for cells and platelets.

Golgi apparatus area of cellular protein packaging.

hematology study of blood and blood-forming tissues in the body.

hemostasis cessation of bleeding.

homeostasis state of normal functioning of the body.

homogeneous of uniform composition.

metabolism all chemical activities needed to produce and utilize cellular energy.

microscope instrument used to view objects not visible to the human eye.

mitochondria cellular organelles that provide energy.

morphology shape of the nucleus, cell, or anatomical structure.

MSDS sheet Material Safety Data Sheet that accompanies chemicals; describes safety features and handling requirements of chemicals.

nosocomial infections infections pertaining to or originating in a health care facility.

nucleus area of the cell where the DNA is found; controls production of proteins within the cytoplasm.

nucleolus area in the nucleus where RNA is synthesized.

organelles parts of a eukaryotic or prokaryotic cell.

OSHA Occupational Safety and Health Administration; governmental agency that regulates many aspects of health and safety protection on the job.

physiology function of a structure or cell within the body.

pluripotent hematopoietic stem cell undifferentiated cell that gives rise to all cell lines found within the bone marrow.

ribosomes packages of RNA where protein synthesis takes place.

spectrophotometer instrument used to detect differences in the amount of light striking a photocell at various wavelengths.

thrombocytes disk-shaped portions of cells used in blood coagulation; also called platelets.

transmittance amount of detectable light passing through a sample.

Universal Precautions list of safety precautions for health care workers published by the Centers for Disease Control and Prevention (CDC).

INTRODUCTION

The study of blood and blood forming tissues is called **hematology**. It is one of many sciences associated with the clinical laboratory science profession. Hematology deals primarily with the **formed elements** of the blood, called cells (see Figure 1.1). There are three types of formed elements:

- red blood cells that carry the oxygen molecules to the body cells for **metabolism**
- white blood cells that form the first line of defense against invasion from microorganisms
- **thrombocytes** that are involved in blood coagulation

The normal and abnormal values of these formed elements and their associated functions make up the fundamentals of hematology. The complex mechanisms associated with the cessation of bleeding (**hemostasis**) is also a part of hematology. Constituents found within the plasma are tested in the chemistry department.

The clinical hematology laboratory represents a challenge to the student. Testing procedures, the complexity of modern instrumentation, and the challenge of blood cell identification in the diagnosis of disease make the department a dynamic environment in which to work. There is always a critical need for adherence to safety rules and regulations.

SAFETY IN THE HEMATOLOGY LABORATORY

Safety issues in the hematology laboratory include:

- being constantly aware of patient safety
- carefully handling potentially pathogenic specimens, complex equipment, and potentially injurious chemicals
- responding appropriately to a laboratory injury and the actions of the laboratory scientist after the injury

It must be the goal of every laboratory scientist to prevent being injured while employed. Safety rules have been implemented by the Occupational Safety and Health Administration (**OSHA**) to assist in this endeavor. However, if injury does occur, procedures have been established to ensure that the health and rights of the individual are protected.

UNIVERSAL PRECAUTIONS

The Centers for Disease Control and Prevention (CDC) in Atlanta, Georgia, has developed a group of **Universal Precautions** that are to be incorporated as part of safety issues for all laboratory departments. These precautions are listed in Exercise 1.

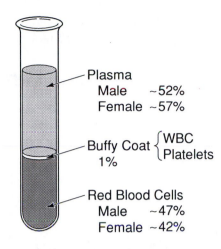

fig. 1.1. Components of blood. (From Marshall. *Fundamental Skills for the Clinical Laboratory Professional.* Delmar, p. 349.)

E X E R C I S E   **UNIVERSAL PRECAUTIONS**

Purpose: To introduce the students immediately to Universal Precautions.

Procedure: Students form small groups of three or four. Discuss each precaution. Determine possible consequences of not following Universal Precautions. Share results with the other groups.

- Consider **ALL** patients' blood and body fluids to be biohazardous.
- Wear latex gloves whenever blood samples are being drawn or when coming in contact with all body fluids, as when performing testing procedures.
- Wash hands when removing gloves or changing gloves between patients or when handling specimens.
- Wear appropriate protection (masks, goggles, gowns, or aprons) if there is a risk of being contaminated.
- All sharp items, such as needles or scalpels, must be placed in puncture-proof containers. Do not bend or break needles.
- Never under any circumstance pipet anything by mouth.
- Clean blood and body fluid spills with a bleach solution or other appropriate hospital disinfectants.
- Immediately report all needle sticks, accidental splashes, wound contamination, or other accidents having to do with bodily fluids.

General safety issues within the hematology laboratory require the student to know the following information contained in Exercise 2.

PERSONNEL SAFETY

Safety procedures should be a part of the daily clinical laboratory routine. There are many important safety habits that the hematologist must adopt to ensure a safe working environment.

EXERCISE   2   **GENERAL SAFETY RULES**

Purpose: To acquaint the student with general rules for safety in the hematology laboratory.

Procedure: Students should be in groups of three or four. The group members should work together to:

LOCATE ALL EXITS—both from the hematology department and from the facility.

LOCATE ALL FIRE EXTINGUISHERS AND FIRE BLANKETS.

LOCATE CHEMICAL SHOWERS AND EYE WASH STATIONS.

DETERMINE IF A SAFETY MANUAL HAS BEEN DEVELOPED FOR THE LABORATORY. Locate it and determine when the last revision was made.

UNDERSTAND THAT THERE ARE STANDARD PROCEDURES TO FOLLOW WHEN COLLECTING SPECIMENS AND PERFORMING TESTS. Locate the procedure manual and familiarize yourself with the contents.

LOCATE THE FUME HOOD. This hood prevents breathing in chemicals that may cause lung damage. It also can protect the laboratory scientist from coming into contact with infectious materials.

LOCATE THE ELECTRICAL FUSE BOX.

INSPECT ANY ELECTRICAL EQUIPMENT FOR WIRING DEFECTS. This will reduce chances of electrocution.

DETERMINE THE REASONS FOR NEVER PLACING HANDS WITHIN ANY WORKING INSTRUMENT OR WEARING JEWELRY WHEN WORKING INSIDE ELECTRICAL INSTRUMENTS. Fingers or limbs could be amputated.

TIE BACK LONG HAIR WHEN TAKING BLOOD OR WORKING IN THE LAB.

LEARN FIRST AID TECHNIQUES AND BE ABLE TO PERFORM CPR IF NECESSARY. Performing emergency first aid could save a life.

REPORT ACCIDENTS ON THE PROPER FORMS TO THE PROPER AUTHORITIES. Make duplicate forms and keep a set for yourself.

Proper Fitting Gloves

Blood and body fluids carry infectious agents. Therefore **GLOVES MUST BE WORN** as prescribed by OSHA standards when handling all specimens. However, gloves do not guard against a needle stick. There is no substitute for proper skill and diligent technique.

Washing the Hands

Unwashed hands can carry many different infectious agents. Hands should be washed frequently in the laboratory, always between glove changes. Upon leaving the laboratory, hands are washed so as not to infect others.

Nosocomial infections are those infections acquired in a hospital setting. They generally occur within 3 days of admission. These hospital-acquired infections can be transmitted by those involved with direct patient care, including laboratory scientists.

Patient Isolation

There are conditions within the hospital setting that require that a particular patient be separated from the general population. This separation is called isolation (see Table 1.1). The equipment necessary to ensure protection varies, depending on the type of infection. The Centers for Disease Control and Prevention (CDC) is directly responsible for developing and relaying the information necessary to deal with isolation procedures. The center has developed new guidelines for a two-tier system, including body substance and specific patient isolation. The body substance isolation is used with all patients and includes Universal Precautions.

Eating, Drinking, or Smoking in the Laboratory

OSHA regulations concerning eating, drinking, and smoking in the laboratory state that a separate area for these activities must be established. They are not to take place in the general laboratory setting. These activities have been shown to

EXERCISE  **LATEX GLOVES THAT FIT**

SAFETY TECHNIQUE: LEARN TO WEAR GLOVES WHEN HANDLING SPECIMENS.

Purpose: To locate and identify the most suitable glove size for each student.

Equipment Needed: Various sizes of latex gloves.

Procedure:
1. Try on all sizes of gloves provided.
2. Look for a glove that fits snugly.
3. Identify the size of the glove by examining the glove box.

EXERCISE **4** **NOSOCOMIAL INFECTIONS**

Purpose: To brainstorm possible sources of nosocomial infections.

Procedure:
1. In small groups (three or four students), list how nosocomial infections can spread throughout a health care facility.
2. Include in the list how laboratory personnel can spread infections, keeping in mind the equipment used to obtain specimens, gloves worn by students, and so on.
3. Share conclusions with other groups about nosocomial infections, identifying actual causes of these infections. Emphasize the importance of handwashing in these conclusions.
4. Invite personnel from the infection control department of a health care facility to comment on student conclusions. Find out what measures infection control departments take to eliminate the spread of infection in their facilities.

Table 1.1. Types of Isolation

Type of Isolation	Possible Reason
Strict isolation	Highly contagious disease
Contact isolation	Scabies infection
Respiratory isolation	Mumps, pertussis, rubella
Drainage precautions	Wound drainage
Tuberculosis isolation	Tuberculosis infection
Enteric precautions	Fecal contamination
Protective or reverse isolation	Protect the patient
Blood/body fluid precautions	Potential contamination from body fluids

open the body to infection. Some chemicals have an additive effect when taken in with food or drink or along with smoke.

Chemicals In The Laboratory
All chemicals in the hematology department are potentially harmful. Labels should be placed on all chemical bottles, with directions for handling each chemical. Labels can also state the need for safety glasses or goggles, a lab coat (with or without an apron), gloves, fume hood, and the various types of fire extinguishers. There is also a coding for the storage of these chemicals. *Blue* signifies a health hazard and should be stored as a poison. *Red* stands for flammability and should be stored in a flammable liquid storage area. *Yellow* represents a reactive hazard and is combustible. *White* indicates a contact hazard and should be stored in a corrosion-proof area. *Orange* labels indicate a chemical with a low rating. These chemicals could be stored in a general chemical storage area.

EXERCISE **5** **PORTALS OF ENTRY**

Purpose: To brainstorm possible invasion of the body through various portals of entry.

Procedure:
1. In small groups (three or four students), list how harmful agents may possibly enter the body.
2. The discussion should include types of agents, what harmful effects can occur, and what portals of entry can be involved.
3. Discuss methods of preventing such infections.
4. Develop a poster showing portals of entry of infection.

EXERCISE **6** **CHEMICAL BOTTLE LABELING**

Purpose: To review the safety labeling of various chemicals.

Equipment Needed: Chemical bottles with manufacturer's labels.

Procedure:
1. In small groups, make a list of the various safety label sections of different chemicals.
2. Be sure to list safety features shown on labels.
3. Note if all chemical bottles have the same information.

Biohazardous Waste Disposal

OSHA regulations also require that laboratories handle biohazardous waste properly. Biohazard bags can be used for body fluid wastes, such as blood tubes and bloody gauze. These bags are purchased already labeled and are sterilized before disposal. Other biohazard wastes, such as chemical wastes, must be collected in special containers and closed and sealed before removal to protect against spillage. The contents of these containers must be labeled properly and handled by a certified waste disposal unit. Figure 1.2 illustrates the universal symbol for biohazardous waste.

Shield Requirements

OSHA also requires that protective shields of acrylic be used when handling open specimens so that aerosol blood products do not contaminate the laboratory. There are various types of shields available, but the most useful type allows for protection without hindering testing.

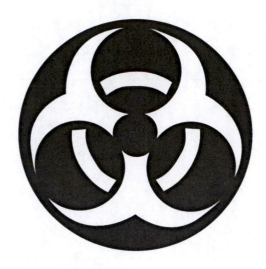

fig. 1.2. Universal symbol for biohazardous waste. (From Flynn/Whitlock. *Clinical Lab Manual Series: Urinalysis.* Delmar.)

E X E R C I S E 7 **BIOHAZARDOUS WASTES**

SAFETY TECHNIQUE: WEAR GLOVES, GOGGLES, MASK IF NECESSARY.

Purpose: To familiarize the student with the proper handling of biohazardous wastes.

Equipment Needed: Biohazard bags (purchased from laboratory supply companies) and chemical biohazard containers (obtain from local biohazard licensed companies).

Procedure:

1. In small groups, make a list of those items in the hematology laboratory that are considered biohazardous.
2. Determine if such items should be placed in biohazard bags or in special containers.
3. Determine which companies in the local area handle biohazards.
4. Find out how these companies dispose of the wastes.

Sharps Containers

A very important safety technique to master concerns sharp instruments such as lancets and needles. Laboratory scientists are continually exposed to sharp objects and are in danger of receiving a puncture wound from one of these instruments. The employer must provide approved containers that can handle

EXERCISE  PROTECTIVE SHIELDS

SAFETY TECHNIQUE: WEAR GLOVES IF HANDLING SPECIMENS.

Purpose: To familiarize the student with protective shields.

Equipment Needed: Several types of protective shields.

Procedure:
1. In small groups, determine which shield best suits the needs of protection while allowing ease in testing.
2. Note that some shields protect better than others, depending on the student involved.
3. Determine if a complete range of motion is available for each student.

sharp instruments and broken glass. The containers are made of hard damage-resistant plastic (Figure 1.3).

Laboratory Coats

The employer must provide laboratory coats for protection of employees. These laboratory coats can be made of disposable paper, cotton, or synthetic fibers. The coats provide protection to employee clothing and can be rapidly removed if a chemical spillage occurs. Laboratory coats are to be removed when employees leave the laboratory for non-work related activities.

Record Keeping

Record keeping must be completed on standard forms and maintained by the laboratory for a prescribed period of time. For example, when an employee is injured, a record must be kept for 30 years after termination of employment.

MSDS Sheets

Material Safety Data Sheets (**MSDS**) are vital to the "right to know" law and the safety in the laboratory. They dictate how chemicals are to be handled, what safety precautions are needed, and how to dispose of wastes properly. These sheets are to be kept for each chemical in the laboratory (Figure 1.4).

ELECTRICAL EQUIPMENT IN THE HEMATOLOGY LABORATORY

The hematologist is constantly using electrical equipment to perform blood counts, differentials, coagulation studies, and so on. There is a continual need for inspection of equipment for possible failure. If problems arise, these should be brought to the attention of the laboratory supervisor.

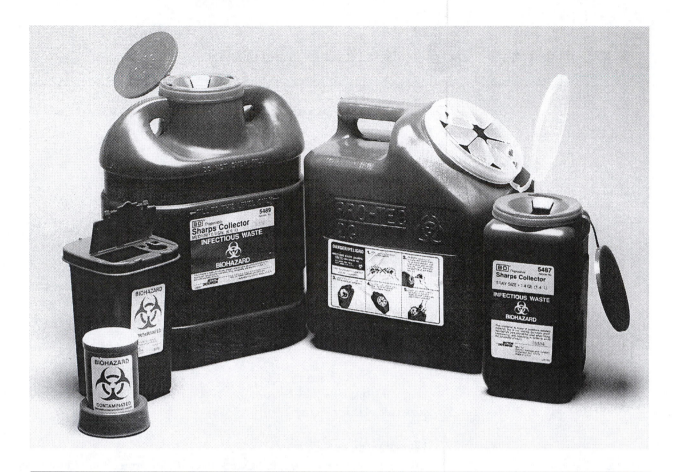

fig. 1.3. Sharp containers. (From Hoeltke. *Phlebotomy.* p. 22.)

E X E R C I S E 9 LABORATORY COATS

Purpose: To discuss the effectiveness of the laboratory coat.

Equipment Needed: Students should be wearing a laboratory coat.

Procedure:
1. In small groups, discuss those instances in which a laboratory coat might provide protection.
2. Discuss the use of buttons or snaps to keep the coat closed. Could there be a problem if a chemical spillage takes place directly on the coat?
3. Determine where laboratory coats should be stored and how often they should be cleaned. How might patients react to bloody, unwashed laboratory coats?

EXERCISE **LABORATORY RECORD KEEPING**

Purpose: To involve the student in determining which records must be kept by the laboratory and for how long.

Equipment Needed: A variety of laboratory records, such as test result records, accident forms, and quality control charts.

Procedure:

1. Using resource materials provided by your instructor, determine which records are required by law to be kept.
2. Using resource materials, find out about accrediting agencies, government regulations and documents, and standards that impact on laboratory record keeping. If necessary, interview laboratory management in a nearby health care facility for more information.
3. What length of time should various records be kept? Can they be kept on a computer disk?

EXERCISE **11** **USING MSDS SHEETS**

Purpose: To prepare students to use safety sheets to help ensure a safe work environment.

Equipment Needed: MSDS sheets from various chemicals found in the hematology laboratory.

Procedure:

1. Obtain MSDS sheets for at least five different chemicals and note the information concerning manufacturer, location of MSDS sheets, emergency telephone number, and any special instructions.
2. Note the following information for each chemical: product identification, physical data, reactivity data, health hazard data, precautionary measures, first aid data, spill and disposal procedures, and transportation data.
3. Note the identification of the manufacturer, what emergency telephone numbers are available, and any warranty waivers.

MATERIAL SAFETY DATA SHEET

For Assistance, Contact:
Regulatory Affairs Dept.
PO Box 907   Ames, IA

HACH COMPANY
PO BOX 907
Ames, IA 50010

Emergency Telephone #
(515) 232-2533

I. PRODUCT IDENTIFICATION

CATALOG NUMBER: 14909
CAS. NO: Not applicable
FORMULA: Not applicable
CHEMICAL FAMILY: Not applicable

PRODUCT NAME: Acetate Buffer Solution
CHEMICAL NAME: Not applicable

II. INGREDIENTS

INGREDIENTS	%	TWA	CAS NUMBER	NATURE of HAZARD	RCRA
Sodium Acetate Trihydrate	<30	None listed	127-09-3	Moderately toxic; may cause irritation	None
Acetic Acid, Glacial	<50	10 ppm	64-19-7	corrosive	None
Demineralized Water	to 100	Not applicable	1732-18-5	None	None

III. PHYSICAL DATA

STATE: liquid | APPEARANCE: Clear, colorless | ODOR: acetic acid

SOLUBILITY IN: WATER: Miscible | ACID: Miscible | OTHER: Not determined

BOILING PT.: 101.5 | MELTING PT.: NA | SPECIFIC GRAVITY: 1.130 | pH: 4.0

VAPOR PRESSURE: Not determined | VAPOR DENSITY (air = 1): ND | EVAPORATION RATE: 0.76

METAL CORROSIVITY—ALUMINUM: None   STEEL: None | SHELF LIFE: stable >1 year

STORAGE PRECAUTIONS: Store tightly closed.

IV. FIRE, EXPLOSION HAZARD AND REACTIVITY DATA

FLASH PT.: >202F; 94.5C | METHOD: closed cup | FLAMMABILITY LIMITS—LOWER: ND   UPPER: ND

SUSCEPTIBILITY TO SPONTANEOUS HEATING: None

SHOCK SENSITIVITY: None | AUTOIGNITION PT.: ND

EXTINGUISHING MEDIA: water, carbon dioxide, or dry chemical

UNUSUAL FIRE AND EXPLOSION HAZARD: May react with oxidizers; may emit toxic fumes

HAZARDOUS DECOMPOSITION PRODUCTS: Toxic fumes of CO_x

OXIDIZER: No | NFPA Codes   Health: 1   Flammability: —   Reactivity: —

CONDITIONS TO AVOID: Heat, flames; contact with oxidizers, sodium peroxide, carbonates, hydroxides, oxides, phosphates

V. HEALTH HAZARD DATA

THIS PRODUCT IS irritating to eyes, skin and respiratory tract.

ACUTE TOXICITY: Moderately toxic
ROUTE OF MOST DETRIMENTAL EXPOSURE: ingestion
TARGET ORGANS: Not determined

CHRONIC TOXICITY: Not determined
ROUTE OF MOST DETRIMENTAL EXPOSURE: Not determined
TARGET ORGANS: Not determined

LONG-TERM EFFECTS: Not applicable
ROUTE OF EXPOSURE: Not applicable
TARGET ORGANS: Not applicable

OVEREXPOSURE: May cause irritation

fig. 1.4. MSDS sheet. (Reprinted with permission from Hach Company.)

Hach Company
WORLD HEADQUARTERS
PO Box 389 Loveland, CO 80539

Hach Europe
BP 51
B5000 Namur 1
Belgium

VI. PRECAUTIONARY MEASURES

Wash thoroughly after handling.
Avoid contact with eyes, skin and clothing.

PROTECTIVE EQUIPMENT: adequate ventilation, safety glasses, disposable gloves

VII. FIRST AID

EYE AND SKIN CONTACT: Immediate flush eyes with water for 15 minutes. Call physician. Flush skin with plenty of water.

INGESTION: Give large quantities of water or milk. Follow with at least 1 ounce of milk of magnesia in an equal amount of water. Induce vomiting by sticking finger down throat. Never give anything by mouth to an unconscious person. Call physician.

INHALATION: Remove to fresh air.

VIII. SPILL AND DISPOSAL PROCEDURES

IN CASE OF SPILL OR RELEASE: Cover contaminated surfaces with soda ash or sodium bicarbonate. Mix and add water if necessary. Scoop up the slurry and wash the neutral waste down the drain with excess water. Wash the site with soda ash solution.

DISPOSE OF IN ACCORDANCE WITH ALL FEDERAL, STATE, AND LOCAL REGULATIONS.

IX. TRANSPORTATION DATA

PROPER SHIPPING NAME: NCR

HAZARD CLASS: Not applicable | ID: NA

DATE: 11/26/85 | CHANGE NO.: 3925

X. REFERENCES

1) In-house information
2) Judgement of technical person compiling data.
3)
4)
5)
6)
7)
8)

THE INFORMATION CONTAINED HEREIN IS BASED ON DATA CONSIDERED ACCURATE. HOWEVER, NO WARRANTY IS EXPRESSED OR IMPLIED REGARDING THE ACCURACY OF THESE DATA OR THE RESULTS TO BE OBTAINED FROM THE USE THEREOF.

fig. 1.4. *(continued)*

FUME HOOD

The fume hood is a piece of equipment with an exhaust fan to keep harmful chemical fumes away from the user.

SPECTROPHOTOMETER

One instrument used in the hematology department as well as other departments in the laboratory is the **spectrophotometer**. It breaks white light into its various wavelengths and projects the individual different colors through an aperture to strike a photoelectric cell. The intensity is registered on a meter, to be read as percent **transmittance** or **absorbance**. Many modern laboratories use this instrument as only a backup instrument. The automated cell counter, the most frequently used instrument in hematology laboratories today, is discussed in Unit 9.

MICROSCOPE

A most useful instrument in the hematology laboratory is the light **microscope,** created by early Danish lens polishers in the seventeenth century. This instrument has been critical in advancing the medical profession to its present state.

In 1663, Robert Hooke established the concept that cells were the basic units of life. His microscopic studies, and those that followed, established the presence

---

E X E R C I S E **12** **USE OF THE FUME HOOD**

SAFETY TECHNIQUE: WEAR GLOVES WHEN HANDLING CHEMICALS AND DRY ICE.

Purpose: To familiarize students with the use of a fume hood.

Equipment Needed: Fume hood, match, soft laboratory tissues, dry ice, water, flowmeter.

Procedure:
1. Stand in front of the fume hood.
2. Turn on the light switch and exhaust fan.
3. Place some dry ice and water under the hood. The smoke from the dry ice and water should be directed toward the exhaust fan.
4. If this is difficult to see, take a soft laboratory tissue and hold it by one corner so that the free side can move toward the exhaust fan. There should be visible movement.
5. These techniques do not illustrate the efficiency of the equipment. To determine this, a flowmeter must be used. This is an instrument that measures airflow in linear feet per minute (fpm). An adequate flow velocity is 60 to 100 fpm, with 100 fpm preferred. Within this range the student can be assured that the fume hood is functioning properly. Take the flowmeter and measure the airflow in the fume hood. Does this comply with the preferred rate?

EXERCISE ▮13▮ THE SPECTROPHOTOMETER

SAFETY TECHNIQUE: WEAR GLOVES; USE CAUTION WHEN WEARING JEWELRY AND HANDLING WIRES.

Purpose: To familiarize the student with the spectrophotometer.

Equipment Needed: A spectrophotometer, strips of white paper about 3 inches long and ½ inch wide, cuvettes.

Procedure:
1. In student pairs, observe and begin to use the spectrophotometer.
2. Note the scale for reading results, the wavelength adjuster, the cuvette holder, the zeroing adjustment, and the transmittance/absorbance control.
3. DO NOT PLUG THE MACHINE INTO THE ELECTRICAL OUTLET.
4. Observe the electrical cord for exposure of copper wire.
5. If the cord is safe, plug the machine into the wall socket.
6. Place a cuvette into the cuvette holder. Turn on the machine.
7. Place a piece of the white paper in the cuvette.
8. Leave the covering off the cuvette. Look down into the cuvette from above.
9. Adjust the wavelength control to the red wavelength range of 650 nm.
10. Adjust the wavelength control toward the violet range by turning the adjustment and observing the color changes on the paper.
11. Note the wavelengths for red, yellow, green, blue, and violet light.

Note: Room lights may have to be off to see the colors clearly. View the colors from the right side of the cuvette holder.

of **organelles** found within the plasma membrane of the cell, all working together to maintain **homeostasis.**

Early physicians were able to note that blood contained many different cells. These physicians gathered data about these cells, describing both their **morphology** and **physiology.**

Utilizing the knowledge gained from various studies, the early hematologists saw white blood cells as belonging to two groups. There were cells that had **filaments** associated with the **nucleus** and those that had a solid nucleus.

It took many years before the maturation of blood cells was clearly understood. Research has shown that blood cells develop from a **pluripotent hematopoietic stem cell.** This unspecialized stem cell is found in the bone marrow and was described by David Golde in the December 1991 issue of *Scientific American*.

In order to observe cells, it is necessary to focus and utilize a binocular microscope, the standard for the hematology field.

EXERCISE 14 THE COMPOUND MICROSCOPE

Purpose: To develop familiarity with the microscope.

Equipment Needed: A compound binocular microscope.

Procedure:

Note: This exercise has general guidelines about a compound microscope. Instructors may find it useful to provide procedures and diagrams that are specific to the microscope model being used by the students.

1. Place the microscope on a bench or table where it can be observed from a side view.
2. Note that the base of the instrument usually has a built-in light source. This light can be adjusted to obtain more or less light. A mirror may be located here to reflect light through the instrument from a separate source.
3. Plug in the instrument and turn it on.
4. Observe the top of the microscope. There are two tubes in which two oculars (eyepieces) are located.
5. Remove one of the oculars and observe it carefully. Numbers followed by the letter "X" are located on the ocular. These indicate that the lens in the ocular magnifies objects by the number on the ocular. If the number is 10X, the magnification of the object is ten times its normal size.
6. Replace the ocular in its tube. Notice that the base of one tube includes ribbing. The base of the other tube is solid. Turn the ribbing and note that the tube moves outward or inward. Most individuals have one strong eye and one weaker eye. The movable tube side is there to respond to these differences.
7. Look between the two eye tubes. See if the microscope has an adjustment wheel that adjusts for the width of the face. Look into both eye tubes and adjust the wheel until only one round light is observed. Take note of any number on the wheel—this is the width of your face.
8. Look along the side of the microscope and identify the adjustment knobs. Usually both knobs are together, with the larger of the two being the coarse adjustment and the smaller being the fine adjustment. Turn the coarse adjustment. Observe the movement of the stage. Now turn the fine adjustment. Is the movement of the stage similar?
9. The part of the microscope moving up and down is called the stage (on some microscopes, the nosepiece moves instead of the stage). Prepared glass slides are placed on the stage.
10. Notice clips that are mounted on the stage. They secure the slides on the stage's surface. Open the movable part and slip in a microscope slide. GENTLY allow the movable part to come in contact with the slide. Make sure the slide is secure.

E X E R C I S E   14   THE COMPOUND MICROSCOPE *(continued)*

11. On the side and under the stage, a set of knobs move the slide holder. Determine which knob moves forward and back. Which knob moves the stage right and left?

12. Above the stage is the revolving nosepiece. It can turn to the left or right. A series of objectives are found attached to the nosepiece and can be changed by unscrewing objectives. The microscope may only have three objectives for use in the hematology department: low, high (sometimes called high dry), and oil immersion. Determine the total magnification of a particular objective by multiplying the nosepiece number by the ocular number.

13. Look directly under the stage to see the cone-shaped condenser with the movable handle for the iris diaphragm. Both of these parts help change the amount of light entering the objective through the stage. Move the condenser up and down. Open and close the iris diaphragm to see what combinations feel acceptable.

14. Use a prepared slide obtained from the instructor to learn the technique of focusing on a slide. **Always start with low power**. After the object is in focus, adjust to high power and then oil immersion. **Caution**: The slide and lenses can be damaged if you try to focus under high power first.

15. When you have finished with the microscope, your instructor will show you how to properly wipe the oil from the oil immersion lens. Some microscopes are covered, put away in a cabinet, or left on the bench in the laboratory. Be sure to follow your instructor's instructions carefully. Forming good habits while working with a microscope can prevent costly service calls.

16. Find out what the routine maintenance schedule is for the microscopes you use. What is done during routine maintenance? What are the most common problems that can occur with a microscope due to a careless user?

Figure 1.5 shows a diagram of the compound light microscope. Be familiar with the name and uses of each part.

There are several types of microscopes available for use within the hematology laboratory. The type just discussed is called the compound light microscope. It has the capability of enlarging specimens about 1000 times their normal size. One limitation encountered with this type of microscope is that the slides are of dead or dying cells. The phase contrast microscope presents the light source from a different angle and can be used to observe living tissue. The magnification with the phase contrast is about the same as for the compound light microscope.

Beyond the magnification of the light microscope is the scanning electron microscope that scans surface features of a specimen treated with a thin layer of

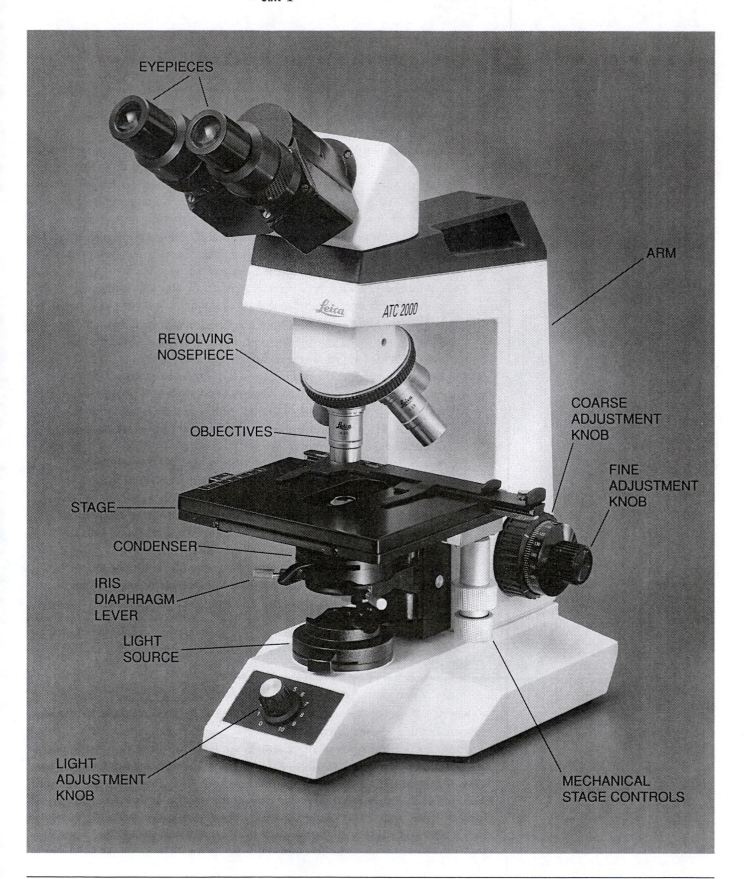

fig. 1.5. Compound microscope. (From Walters. *Basic Medical Laboratory Techniques.* ed. 3. p. 82.)

E X E R C I S E  **TYPES OF MICROSCOPES**

Purpose: To research various types of microscopes.

Procedure:
1. List the types of microscopes presently available and their respective magnification ranges.
2. Using the same list, determine the feasibility of using each microscope in the hematology laboratory.
3. Discuss with your instructor the various types of inserts that are utilized in hematology to create restricted fields, filters used to enhance inclusion bodies, and additional types of calculations necessary to determine magnification, working distance, and so on.

E X E R C I S E **16** **OBSERVING WHITE BLOOD CELL MORPHOLOGY**

Purpose: To identify white blood cell morphology.

Equipment Needed: Microscope and slides provided by the instructor.

Procedure:
1. Sit in front of the microscope and adjust the chair to achieve a comfortable sitting position.
2. Take the prepared slide provided and hold it up to a light source. Observe the edge of the blood smear where the blood is the lightest. This is called the *feathered edge*. The microscope objective is to be focused in this area.
3. Place the prepared slide on the stage and secure it in place using the movable arm.
4. Focus under low power to find an area where the cells are just touching each other.
5. Turn the revolving nosepiece half way between the low power and oil immersion objective and place a drop of oil directly onto the slide.
6. Now click the oil immersion objective into place. Using the fine adjustment, focus on the cells on the prepared slide.
7. Adjust the light source to increase the amount of light for this higher magnification.
8. Make a drawing of the microscope field.

9. Notice that the most common round cell in the field of vision has no dark staining nucleus. These are the red blood cells, which are about 7.0 µ in diameter with a thin central area.

10. Move the slide on the stage using the adjustment knobs, looking for a larger cell with a purple staining nucleus. This is a white blood cell. It is called *white* because many cells together form a whitish layer above the red blood cells in a typical blood tube if left to stand for a period of time. Make a drawing of these cells. Note the variety of white blood cells found.

11. *Neutrophils* are about 13 µm (micrometers) in diameter and generally have three lobes to their nuclear material, all connected by filaments. Use the fine adjustment to see the filaments. Observe the cytoplasm of the cells. Notice the granulation in the cytoplasm. These cells are the most common white blood cell type, making up 50% to 70% of the white blood cells seen.

12. *Lymphocytes* are smaller, with a solid nucleus. This is the second most common cell, making up about 20% to 35% of the white cells seen. These cells may or may not have visible cytoplasm.

13. *Monocytes* are the largest white blood cells in peripheral circulation. The diameter is about 12 to 30 µm. A large lobular nucleus is seen in a grayish cytoplasm. They make up about 2% to 6% of the total white blood cells seen.

14. Scan the feathered end of the slide for a cell with large red/orange or purple/black granules covering it. These cells are the rarer white blood cells. The reddish cell is an *eosinophil*, making up 0% to 3% of the white blood cells seen. The purplish is a *basophil*, making up about 0% to 1% of the white blood cells seen.

15. Look for some very small blobs of purple-red material between the red cells. These are platelets, utilized in coagulation of blood.

16. The typical white blood cell has many parts. The morphology of each type of cell is used to classify them. Make as many drawings as necessary to illustrate the various types of white cells seen on the slides provided by the instructor.

Note: Extremely valuable resources to aid in identification of white blood cells are color plates of white blood cells, found in many hematology reference manuals.

metal. The transmission electron microscope is the most powerful instrument available today, magnifying to several hundred thousand times normal size.

White blood cells have a circular area that stains darker than the rest of the cell. This area is usually more condensed and **homogeneous** and is the site of cellular control. This part of the cell is called the **nucleus** where the DNA, in the form of **chromatin**, is found. Within the nucleus may be seen a smaller circular or oblong lighter staining area. This is the **nucleolus**, where a type of RNA is found and used by the cell to make proteins. The presence of nucleoli indicates metabolically active cells. White blood cells that are metabolically active are restricted to very early forms found in the bone marrow.

Surrounding the nucleus is a thin halo that may not stain at all. This is where the **Golgi apparatus** is found. The Golgi apparatus is the packaging plant of the cell. Proteins made on the **ribosomes** are packaged in vacuoles that eventually circulate throughout the cell.

The **cytoplasm** is all the material inside the cell composed of water and dissolved chemicals. With special staining, the **mitochondria** can be seen. They are the powerhouses of the cell. The cytoplasm can have granules that stain with specific vital stains. These are vacuoles created by the Golgi apparatus and have specific functions in the cell. The granules in eosinophils pick up the acid stain eosin, resulting in red to orange granules. The granules in basophils pick up the basic stain methylene blue, resulting in blue to black granules.

The cell has channels that help distribute chemicals throughout the cytoplasm called the **endoplasmic reticulum.** If this network of channels is associated with ribosomes, it is called rough endoplasmic reticulum. If there are no ribosomes attached to the endoplasmic reticulum, it is called smooth endoplasmic reticulum.

Most of the organelles described above are seen only with special staining procedures or with the transmission electron microscope (Figure 1.6).

E X E R C I S E **THE CELLULAR NUCLEUS AND NUCLEOLUS**

Purpose: To demonstrate various types of cell nuclei and nucleoli.

Equipment Needed: Prepared slides provided by the instructor.

Procedure:
1. Observe the prepared slide for the feathered edge. This will be the area of focus.
2. Place the prepared slide on the stage, securing it in place using the movable arm.
3. Focus under low power to find an area where the cells are just touching each other.
4. Turn the revolving nosepiece halfway between the low power and oil immersion objective. Place a drop of oil directly onto the slide.
5. Click the oil immersion objective into place. Using the fine adjustment, focus on the cells on the prepared slide.
6. Adjust the light source to increase the amount of light for this higher magnification.
7. Find a white blood cell and identify it. Check the identification with your instructor.
8. Find the nucleus and observe for the nucleolus.
9. Draw your findings.

E X E R C I S E   **18**   **EOSINOPHILIC AND BASOPHILIC GRANULES**

Purpose: To reacquaint the student with these cells, specifically viewing cellular granules.

Equipment Needed: Microscope and prepared slides provided by the instructor.

Procedure:

1. Repeat steps 1 to 7 of Exercise 16.
8. Observe for red- to orange-staining granules in the cytoplasm of a white blood cell.
9. Make a drawing of this eosinophil, observing and drawing the granules as accurately as possible.
10. Observe for blue- to black-staining granules in the cytoplasm of a white blood cell.
11. Make a drawing of this basophil, observing and drawing the granules as accurately as possible.

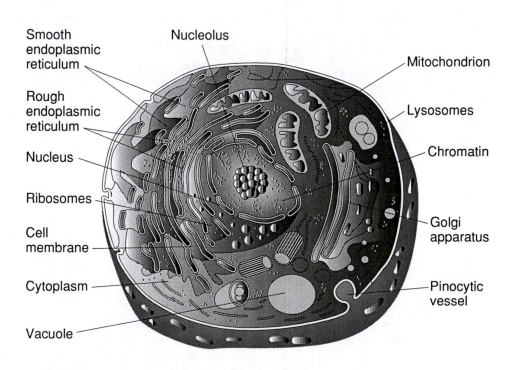

fig. 1.6. Fine structure of an animal cell. (From Fong's *Microbiology for Health Careers.* ed. 5. Delmar 1994, p. 68.)

SUMMARY

Hematology is the study of blood and blood-forming tissues of the human body. Specifically, hematology focuses on the formed elements of the blood called cells. There are three types of formed elements in the blood: red blood cells, white blood cells, and thrombocytes (platelets). The normal and abnormal values of these elements and their associated functions make up the fundamentals of hematology.

Testing procedures, complexity of modern instrumentation, and the blood cell identification challenges present a need for adherence to safety rules and regulations within the hematology department. Universal Precautions have been developed by the Centers for Disease Control and Prevention (CDC) to make the health care environment as safe as possible when dealing with patients' blood and body fluids. Understanding how to prevent the spread of infection (wearing proper gloves, washing hands frequently and properly, and so on) is crucial when working in the laboratory environment.

Handling chemicals in the laboratory in a safe fashion, disposing of biohazardous waste properly, and being aware of potential electrical hazards in the laboratory are all a part of ensuring a safe work environment. Proper record keeping in the laboratory, including the storage of test result records, accident forms, and quality control charts, is an integral part of maintaining high standards of performance in the laboratory.

The proper use and maintenance of instruments in the hematology laboratory is another critical part of maintaining a safe, well-functioning hematology department. The compound microscope is the most important instrument used in this department, and competence must be gained in using the microscope, as the hematologist must be capable of recognizing and identifying accurately all blood cells.

REVIEW QUESTIONS

1. Hematology is the science that deals primarily with
   a. hemoglobin, the red color of blood
   b. the formed elements of the blood
   c. the origin of the plasma
   d. all of the above
2. The blood plasma constitutes what percentage of normal blood?
   a. 22%
   b. 45%
   c. 55%
   d. 80%

3. Food and vitamins are associated with which component of the blood?
   a. plasma proteins
   b. leukocytes and thrombocytes
   c. erythrocytes
   d. other solutes

4. Of the following, which is NOT one of the Universal Precautions?
   a. wear latex gloves when handling specimens
   b. place all sharp items in a puncture-proof container
   c. when pipetting by mouth, use safety pipets
   d. wear appropriate protection if there is a risk of contamination

5. What are nosocomial infections?
   a. infections that are life threatening
   b. infections passed from one individual to another
   c. infections that cannot be treated with antibiotics
   d. infections often occurring within 3 days of hospital admission

6. All chemicals are potentially harmful. Which of the following is the label color for a health hazard?
   a. blue
   b. red
   c. yellow
   d. white
   e. orange

7. Information concerning the handling safety of chemicals is called
   a. a package label
   b. an MSDS sheet
   c. a special instruction sheet
   d. all of the above

8. What is the prescribed velocity for a chemical fume hood?
   a. 30 to 40 fpm
   b. 40 to 60 fpm
   c. 60 to 100 fpm
   d. 0 to 100 fpm

9. The magnification power of the compound microscope is calculated by
   a. multiplying the ocular power by the objective power
   b. adding the ocular power and the objective power
   c. multiplying the low objective power by the high objective power
   d. adding all objective powers together

10. The portion of the cell responsible for the control of the cell is the
    a. Golgi apparatus
    b. nucleus
    c. ribosome
    d. nucleolus

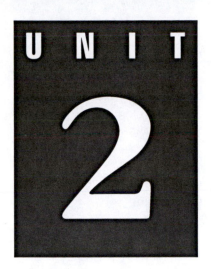

UNIT 2

Measurement in the Hematology Laboratory

Having completed this unit, it is the responsibility of the student to know the following:

- Calculate the mean, median, and range of a set of test scores.

- Calculate and define the standard deviation of a set of test scores.

- Graph the results of test scores on a histogram.

- Interpret the results of the above calculations and graph.

- Apply the results of the calculations and graphs to a quality control program.

GLOSSARY

accuracy measuring the "true" components of a sample.

diurnal having a daily cycle.

Gaussian distribution another name for a normal bell-shaped curve, where the distribution of values are plotted around the mean.

histogram visual representation of a population's data.

mean average score in a set of test results.

median exact middle score in a set of test results.

mode most common score in a set of test results.

precision repeated test scores regardless of accuracy.

skewed distribution graphic representation obtained when special factors are altering the results.

standard deviation a measure of the spread of a values population around the mean.

Westgard's rules set of guidelines to determine when a method is out of control.

INTRODUCTION

Statistical analysis is utilized in the hematology laboratory as a means of determining the normal values for a particular test procedure. Statistics are also used in the analysis of quality control information. Without calculating the differences in a sample population, the relationships among the sample population cannot be determined. This requires that the student have a basic knowledge of statistics.

RANGE

The following exercise will develop the skill needed to determine the range of a set of test scores. The range is the determination of the most extreme scores. The range illustrates the spread of scores. However, it does not predict what the dispersion of scores will be like in the future. It is offered as a means of beginning statistical analysis.

E X E R C I S E  CALCULATION OF RANGE

Purpose: The calculation of the range of a set of test results enables the hematologist to determine extremes in a set of test results.

Equipment Needed: Paper, pencil, and the sets of scores.

Procedure:
1. Below are three sets of different test scores. Each set of scores is to be treated independently. The student should copy each set of scores on a different piece of paper in descending order.
2. Once the scores are arranged on the paper look for the highest score in the set and also the lowest score in the set. This is the RANGE of the set of scores. Do not discard the results.

Set One			Set Two			Set Three		
5000	3500	4500	12.0	13.0	12.5	50	45	35
7500	4000	6500	11.5	14.2	15.0	39	47	42
6350	5000	7000	9.0	10.8	13.5	36	39	38
5500	5900	6200	11.0	10.6	12.5	42	45	32
3000	6500	8000	14.0	15.0	11.9	30	40	47

MEAN

The mean is the average of the test scores. It is one of the best methods of illustrating a central tendency. Calculating the mean of a set of scores yields the average score for that set of scores only. It is the population mean that is significant in making predictions about the entire population.

Note that the symbol "Σ" represents the word "sum" and requires that the sum of the individual scores be achieved. This sum is then divided by the number of scores in the sample.

E X E R C I S E **20** **CALCULATION OF MEAN**

Purpose: To develop the skills necessary to calculate the mean.

Equipment Needed: Listed scores and a calculator.

Procedure:
1. Add up all test results below.
2. Divide by the number of tests performed. You have calculated the average score, called the **mean** by using the formula $\overline{X}$ (pronounced X-bar) = $\sum \dfrac{x}{n}$

10,500	5750	9250	4500	7250	7500	8000	7500	7250	7750
7750	7500	7500	9250	5750	7000	8000	7000	7750	7250

E X E R C I S E **21** **OBTAINING MEANS OF VARIOUS SAMPLES**

Purpose: To increase the student's ability to calculate the mean of various sets of test scores.

Equipment Needed: Sets of scores found in Exercise 19, pencil, and paper.

Procedure:
1. Treat each set of scores independently.
2. Calculate the mean of each set of scores.
3. Do not discard these results, as they will be used in the following procedures.

HISTOGRAM

It is often easier to visually observe the data in the form of a histogram. This requires that the scores be arranged in such a fashion that identical scores are located next to each other (or a hashmark is used).

Look at the representation of the test results in Exercise 22. Draw a line connecting the result listed on the far right. The diagram is a graphic representation of the data. The use of this graphic technique is referred to as developing a **histogram**. It is one of the best ways to visualize data. It can be used to identify the mean, median, and mode scores. If all three scores are the same, a normal population is indicated. Normal populations are represented by a bell-shaped curve called a **Gaussian distribution** (Figure 2.1).

SKEWED DISTRIBUTIONS

Histograms sometimes indicate that other factors are altering test results. When this happens, it is called a **skewed distribution**. When the test results seem to be located around either of the extreme scores, it does not yield a normal distribution. Another alteration in the histogram could be the development of two curves, slightly overlapping each other. This indicates that two different populations were surveyed, such as a male and female population, or an adult and child population. To illustrate these types of curves, perform Exercise 23.

MEDIAN

Another calculation associated with central tendencies is the **median.** It is defined as the exact middle score in a set of test results. To obtain the median, test scores are arranged in descending order. Beginning with the highest score, count the number of scores present. Then divide that number by 2 and count

E X E R C I S E **DEVELOPMENT OF A HISTOGRAM**

Purpose: Detect the mean by arranging the scores in a histogram.

Equipment Needed: The scores from Exercises 19 and 20.

Procedure:
1. Treat the test results from Exercises 19 and 20 independently.
2. Take the individual test results from Exercise 20. Arrange them in a descending order, placing identical results next to each other to indicate the frequency of that score.
3. Repeat this technique for the three sets of results in Exercise 19.

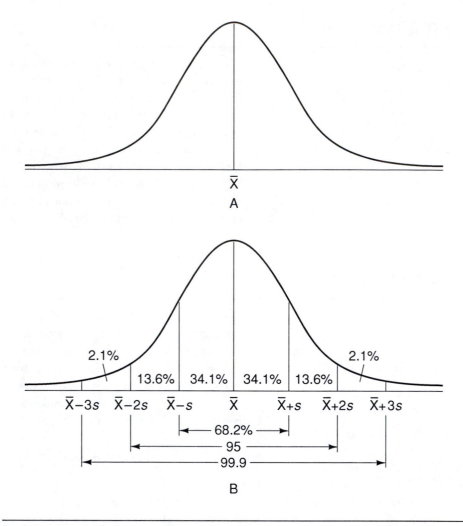

$\overline{X}$

A

B

fig. 2.1. Normal distribution curves. (From Walters. *Basic Medical Laboratory Techniques*, ed. 3. Delmar, 1995, p. 177.)

down from the highest score to the product of the calculation. For example, if there are twenty scores, count down from the highest score to the tenth score below it. That is the median.

MODE

The **mode** is the most frequent score in the set of test scores. Determine the mode for the sets of scores in Exercises 19 and 20.

The mean, median, and mode scores are the same for the data of Exercise 20. The result is a normal curve or Gaussian distribution (Figure 2.1).

STANDARD DEVIATION

A calculation that is an important part of a quality control program is the **standard deviation.** The standard deviation is a measure of the scatter of sam-

EXERCISE **23** SKEWED POPULATIONS

Purpose: To familiarize the student with different types of histograms.

Equipment Needed: Scores listed below, pencil, and paper.

Procedure:
1. Develop a histogram for each set of test scores listed below:

Set One			Set Two			Set Three		
9250	9000	7500	5250	5000	4500	9000	8000	8500
8750	9000	5000	6500	5500	5000	5750	6250	5000
6000	9250	9000	8000	6000	5000	7500	8000	4500
8750	9250	5500	5250	7500	5250	5250	5500	5500
6250	8250	6500	8750	5750	7000	8000	5500	6000

EXERCISE  CALCULATION OF THE MEDIAN

Purpose: To determine the median score value in the sets of scores.

Equipment Needed: Sets of scores from Exercises 19 and 20, pencil, and paper.

Procedure:
1. With the scores arranged in descending order in Exercise 19, count the number of tests in the set.
2. Divide the number received by 2.
3. Count down from the highest score until the product of the division is reached. This is the median.
4. Repeat steps 1 to 3 on the sets of scores in Exercise 20.

ple values around the mean (average) value. Once the mean is determined for a sample of values, the determination can then be made of what is an acceptable variation. When a sample of values is plotted on a graph, the distribution forms a Gaussian curve. In a normal distribution, half of the values are greater than the mean and half are less than the mean.

Once the mean has been determined for a group of values, the standard deviation of the analysis can be calculated. The standard deviation (s or SD) is a measurement of the variation of any single result from the mean or the spread of any obtained value from the mean. Exercise 26 utilizes the test scores given in Exercise 20. Many of today's automated hematology instruments calculate the standard deviation of test values for the laboratory scientist.

E X E R C I S E   **25**   **CALCULATION OF THE MODE**

Purpose: To determine the mode score in a set of test scores.

Equipment Needed: Test values listed in Exercises 19 and 20.

Procedure:
1. Observe the test scores in Exercise 19. Identify the most frequent score. This is the mode score.
2. Repeat for the sets of scores in Exercise 20.

E X E R C I S E   **26**   **CALCULATION OF STANDARD DEVIATION**

Purpose: To familiarize the student with calculating standard deviation.

Equipment Needed: Values from Exercise 20: 10,500 9250 9250 8000 8000 7750 7750 7750 7500 7500 7500 7500 7250 7250 7250 7000 7000 5750 5750 4500, and a calculator.

      The calculated mean for this set of scores was 7500. The range is from 10,500 to 4500, a difference of 6000.

Procedure:
1. Place all of the scores in order as shown above.
2. Subtract the mean from the individual scores and list.
3. Square the results (this eliminates negative numbers because a minus times a minus equals a plus score).
4. Add the scores together.
5. Divide by the number of scores minus one.
6. Take the square root of this sum. This is the standard deviation. The formula for this calculation is:

$$\text{S.D.} = \sqrt{\Sigma\, \frac{(X - \overline{X})^2}{N - 1}}$$

S = 1 standard deviation
Σ = sum of
$\overline{X}$ = mean
X = any observed value
N = total number of observed values

Once the standard deviation has been calculated, it is possible to go back to the Gaussian curve and actually make the percent divisions in it as shown in Figure 2.1, B. This shows that in a normal population 68.2% of all results obtained will fall between 1 SD below the mean and 1 SD above the mean. Additionally, 95.4% of the values will fall between 2 SD below the mean and 2 SD above the mean. If 3 SD are used, 99.6% of all values will fall in this division.

Factors that can influence normal ranges include:

- ethnic origins of patients
- gender
- age
- time of day testing was performed (some results change on an hourly or daily basis, showing a **diurnal** pattern)
- geographical location of sample

QUALITY ASSURANCE IN THE HEMATOLOGY LABORATORY

The clinical laboratory scientist is responsible for the identification of possible errors in test results and for assuring accuracy and precision of results. To achieve this goal, quality assurance in the laboratory is accomplished by bringing together the members of the staff and developing a plan. It includes decreasing errors in **accuracy** and **precision**. It also includes the use of control samples to be tested as if they were patient samples. (Refer to Figure 2.2.)

Laboratory errors can occur anywhere, jeopardizing patient care. These errors can be random, possibly caused by mislabeling a specimen or a transcription error. The error may be systematic, possibly caused by improperly calibrating an instrument or by refrigerators and dry baths not maintaining their temperature. These errors must be eliminated to ensure the best possible test results.

E X E R C I S E  **NORMAL RANGE OF A SAMPLE POPULATION**

Purpose: To illustrate the normal range of the scores from Exercise 20.

Equipment needed: Standard deviation results from Exercise 26, the calculated mean results from Exercise 20, pencil, and paper.

Procedure:
1. Take the calculated mean results and add to it 1 calculated standard deviation result from Exercise 26.
2. Now subtract 1 standard deviation result from the mean.
3. Double the standard deviation result and add to the mean.
4. Double the standard deviation result and subtract from the mean.
5. Steps 3 and 4 calculate the normal range.

ACCURACY AND PRECISION

Laboratory testing should reflect an **accurate** picture of the physiology within the patient's body. To be sure that the results are accurate, the laboratory scientist performs quality control (QC) testing. A control sample is purchased from a manufacturer and then tested as if it were an unknown patient. The results obtained are compared with the target value assigned by the manufacturer. If these results are within 2 standard deviations of the target value, they are within the control limits. They are then plotted on a daily log sheet called a Levey-Jennings chart (Figure 2.3). This chart provides a graphic representation of the confidence level of the results. It can also show any trends toward being out of control, which may indicate contamination of reagents, equipment failure, or employee inaccuracies.

Quality control in the laboratory is required by all certifying agencies to provide the public with standards of practice. Using the mean and standard deviation yields the acceptable normal range of values for each laboratory. When a new test is introduced in the laboratory, the test must be run on significant numbers of the population that is served by the laboratory. Quality control of equipment, including refrigerators and dry baths, normally includes temperature readings and readings of standards, all plotted on Levey-Jennings charts to ensure normal functioning.

The term *accurate* means that the results given to the physician are a true picture of the patient's physiology. The term *precision* means that the same results have been achieved on repeated testing. Precision does not indicate that these results are accurate. The tests performed must also be sensitive enough to detect the unknown value, but not so sensitive as to cloud that value with extraneous data (see Figure 2.1).

In the Levey-Jennings charts depicted in Figure 2.3, a normal variation within 2 standard deviations is illustrated in the top chart. A trend from days 13 through 16 in the lower chart reveals a problem. The laboratory scientist must determine what the problem is and correct it.

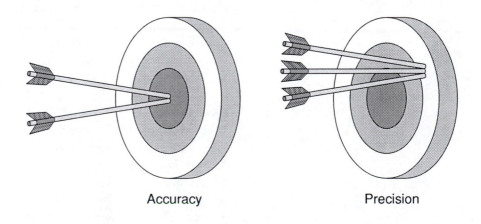

Accuracy   Precision

fig. 2.2. Accuracy and precision. Illustration by Lora Russell.

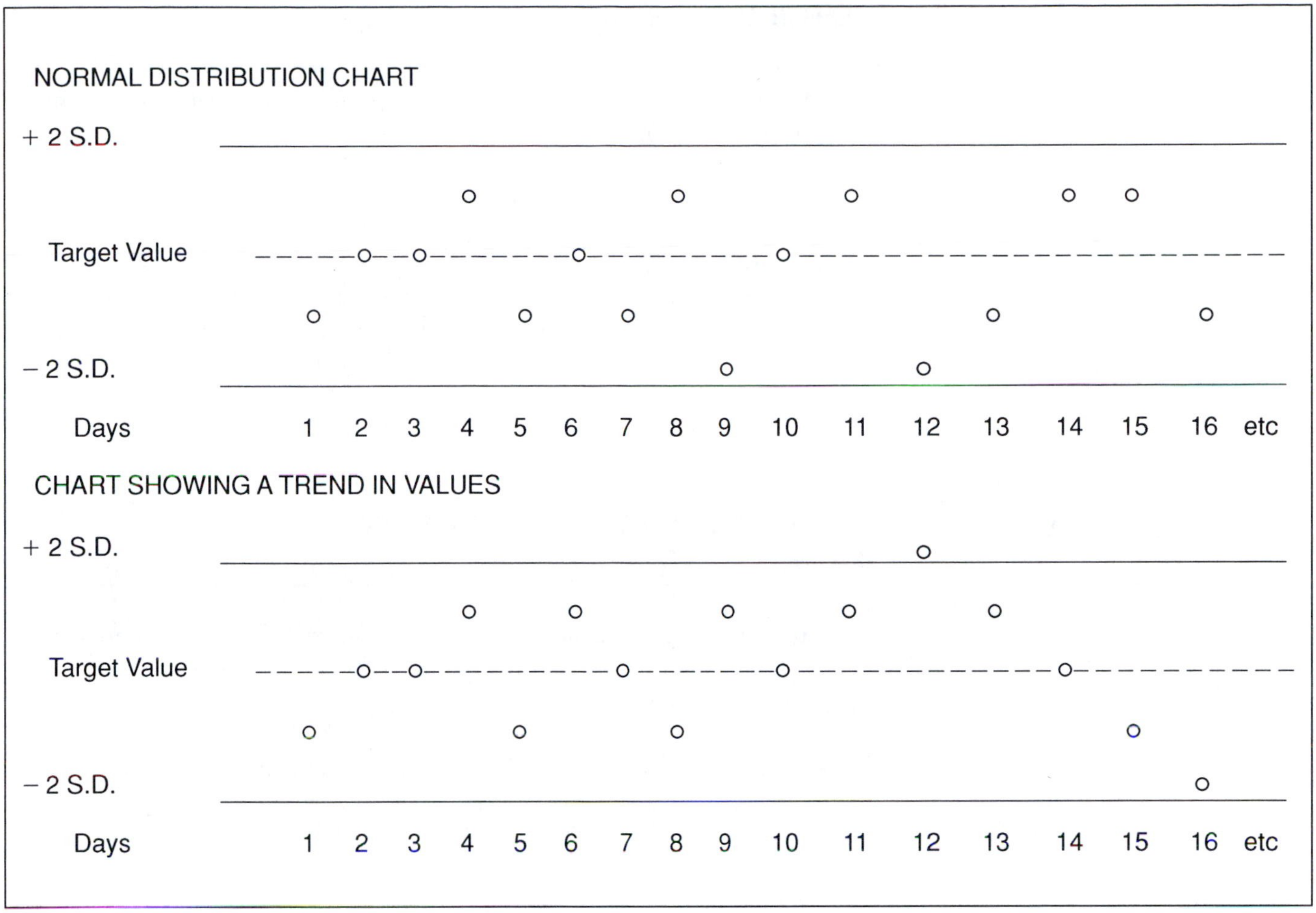

NORMAL DISTRIBUTION CHART

CHART SHOWING A TREND IN VALUES

fig. 2.3. Levey-Jennings chart.

WESTGARD'S RULES

Westgard's rules are a set of rules that provide guidelines for the laboratory scientist to decide whether or not a testing method is out of control. These rules give specific limits about how much error is allowed in the control values before patient test results are rejected.

To utilize these rules, the laboratory must run at least two control sera of different concentrations in every run of patient samples. The run is considered out of control if any of the following occur:

- Both controls are outside the ±2 SD limit.
- One control is outside the ±2 SD limit in two successive runs.
- Controls in four consecutive runs have values greater than ±1 SD, all in the same direction.
- Ten consecutive control values fall either above or below the established mean.

COEFFICIENT OF VARIATION

The coefficient of variation (CV) is a statistic that illustrates the standard deviation as a percentage. It is calculated by dividing the standard deviation by the mean and multiplying by 100 as illustrated by this formula.

$$CV\% = s/\overline{x} \times 100$$

It is used primarily in quality control procedures where the results of a particular level of control concentration are compared over several months to determine the precision of the test method. Usually several control levels are graphed together on a single sheet to illustrate the instruments and test methods performance on a month-to-month basis.

E X E R C I S E   **28**   **COEFFICIENT OF VARIATION**

Purpose: The graphic illustration of several coefficients of variation will yield a means of determining the precision of the testing method.

Equipment Needed: Graph paper, pencil, and the following CVs:

1.0%	1.5%	1.2%	1.0%	2.0%	1.8%	1.0%
1.3%	1.2%	1.0%	1.2%	1.0%		

Procedure:
1. Set up the graph paper with equidistant months of the year on the bottom line.
2. On the left side of the graph, place percentage CVs equidistant as 0.5%, 1.0%, 1.5%, 2.0%, 2.5%, 3.0%.
3. Plot the listed CVs using the first score as the score for January, the second for February, and so on.

SUMMARY

There are many basic statistical procedures that enable the clinical laboratory scientist to obtain useful information about the accuracy of test results. The calculation of range, mean, median, mode, standard deviation, and the development of a histogram are important statistical tools in the hematology laboratory. Graphic representations of data include the histogram and the Levey-Jennings chart.

Quality control testing in the hematology laboratory is critical to maintaining a department that produces reliable results. Laboratory errors can occur anywhere, jeopardizing patient care. Errors can be random, or they can be systematic. All types of error must be eliminated to ensure the best possible test results.

Accuracy is achieved when the *true* value of the sample is measured. Precision is accomplished when test scores yield the same results when repeatedly tested. Accuracy and precision are important concepts in a quality control program. The Levey-Jennings chart yields a way of observing the reliability of results. Quality control monitoring of equipment can be plotted on these charts to assure normal functioning.

Westgard's rules are a set of rules that provide guidelines for deciding whether or not a testing method is out of control. The coefficient of variation is also a useful statistic that illustrates the standard deviation as a percentage.

REVIEW QUESTIONS

1. Identify the mean of the following set of scores: 6, 5, 3, 2, 8, 5, 4, 6, 5, 7
   a. 4.5
   b. 5.1
   c. 6.1
   d. 4.8
2. In the above set of scores, identify the median
   a. 4
   b. 5
   c. 6
   d. 3
3. In the above set of scores, identify the mode
   a. 3
   b. 4
   c. 5
   d. 6
4. Having calculated the above three results, what can be predicted?
   a. a normal distribution occurs
   b. a distribution skewed to the left occurs
   c. a distribution skewed to the right occurs
   d. a bimodal curve occurs

5. Westgard's rules provide guidelines to
   a. identify the standard deviation of results
   b. calculate the coefficient of variation
   c. help decide whether or not a testing method is out of control
   d. none of the above

6. The median represents
   a. the most numerous score
   b. the most extreme score above the mean
   c. the exact middle score
   d. the most extreme score below the mean

7. The average score is the
   a. standard deviation
   b. median
   c. mode
   d. mean

8. The mode represents
   a. the most numerous score
   b. the average
   c. the exact middle score
   d. the most extreme score above the mean

UNIT 3

Blood Cell Counting

LEARNING OBJECTIVES

Having completed this unit, it is the responsibility of the student to know the following:

- Discuss the process for preparing differential slides.

- Describe and perform techniques for counting red and white blood cells.

- Identify the techniques used to count increased numbers of cells.

- Identify the techniques used to count decreased numbers of cells.

- Discuss the various types of hemacytometers and the formulas associated with their use.

- Accurately perform a Wright's stain for a differential cell count.

GLOSSARY

anticoagulant agent that prevents blood coagulation; most are chemicals to which calcium ions attach (citrate, EDTA).

differential count name for slide made in hematology for laboratory scientist to identify and count 100 white blood cells.

EDTA ethylenediaminetetraacetic acid, an anticoagulant found in the lavender-topped tubes used to collect blood; most common anticoagulated blood used in hematology testing as it also preserves cells well.

hemacytometer precision engraved slide used for counting various types of cells.

hematocrit packed cell volume expressed as a percent.

hemoglobin measurement of hemoglobin concentration expressed in grams/dl.

heparin chemical that acts as an anticoagulant.

lyse to break apart.

Neubauer precision ruling of a hemacytometer in common use.

platelet count procedure to count the number of cell fragments (platelets) broken from large cells called megakaryocytes; chief role of the platelet is to aid in blood clotting.

RBC indices red blood cell indices; calculations that determine the size and content of hemoglobin and red blood cells, including the MCV (mean cell volume), MCH (mean cell hemoglobin), and MCHC (mean cell hemoglobin concentration).

INTRODUCTION

The objective of every clinical laboratory scientist is to assist the attending physician in the diagnosis of patient disease and to aid in the surveillance of the effectiveness of the treatment plan. These objectives are accomplished by performing laboratory tests in an effective, thorough, and accurate manner.

One of the most commonly ordered laboratory tests is the complete blood count (CBC). In most cases, the CBC consists of a white blood count (WBC), red blood count (RBC), a **hematocrit** (Hct, a packed cell volume), a **hemoglobin** level (Hb or Hgb), **red blood cell (RBC) indices** (MCV, MCH, MCHC), a **platelet count** (PLTC), and a **differential count** (diff). These tests are presently performed on automated equipment in most clinical laboratories. Laboratory scientists should learn manual methods associated with each test in case of equipment failure (some modern laboratories have automated backup as well). The automated techniques are evaluated in Unit 9.

SAMPLE PREPARATION FOR ANALYSIS

The most common blood sample taken for blood cell counts is the lavender-stoppered tube. This tube contains the **anticoagulant EDTA.** This anticoagulant requires that the tube be inverted several times after drawing the blood to mix the EDTA thoroughly with the blood (phlebotomy techniques are covered in Hoeltke's *Phlebotomy Manual* in this series).

Between the time the blood is drawn and tested, formed elements (cells) may start to settle in the bottom of the tube. Most laboratories are equipped with test tube rotators, as illustrated in Figure 3.1, which will continue to rotate and mix the samples. This will ensure a normal distribution of cells in the plasma.

THE DIFFERENTIAL SLIDE

The EDTA tube drawn for the CBC will provide a blood sample that is put through a cell-counting instrument. Additionally, many laboratories require that a few drops of blood from the EDTA container be put on a slide for microscopic observation, preparing a differential slide. The differential slide is then stained carefully. Information gained from viewing the slide includes obtaining the percentage of each of the five types of leukocytes, determining the morphology of red blood cells and platelets, determining whether or not abnormal immature blood cells are present, and identifying abnormal inclusion bodies in the cells.

Many modern laboratories do not prepare differential slides on all blood samples since the automated blood cell count provides enough information. However, it is important to note that the manual differential provides information that a computerized differential could not, such as specific red cell morphology, platelet morphology, and presence of inclusion bodies. When a physician expects abnormal populations of cells, a differential slide is made to view the cells individually under the microscope. When any results are abnormal in the automated cell count, a differential slide is often made.

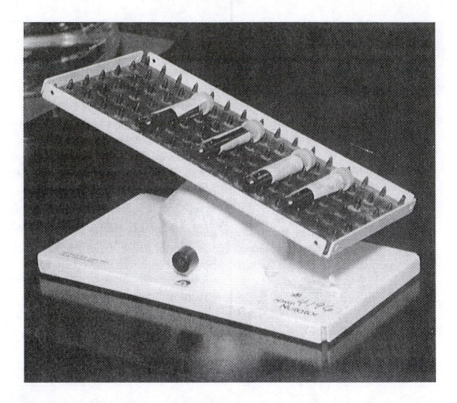

fig. 3.1. Rotator. (From Marshall. *Fundamental Skills for the Clinical Laboratory Professional.* p. 348.)

It takes practice to prepare a differential slide for examination under a microscope. Many students find it difficult to obtain the perfect slide on the first try. Utilizing the techniques found in Exercise 29 should produce slides that can be easily viewed under the microscope for cellular components. Staining techniques will be discussed later in this unit.

Once the technique of making a readable smear has been mastered, the differential count will be much easier to complete. Physicians rely on the laboratory to accurately identify the different types of white blood cells on the differential slide. The technique of reading the differential smear will be discussed in Unit 4.

Between the time the slide is made and read, the clinical laboratory scientist performs other tests on the blood sample. These tests include counting of the various types of cells, performing hematocrit and hemoglobin testing, and calculating the red blood cell indices.

WHITE BLOOD CELL COUNT

The counting of white blood cells (WBCs) gives the physician much usable information for the diagnosis of patient conditions. The number of white blood cells often increases as disease states progress. Therefore, an accurate counting of the white blood cells in a known volume is used to determine the presence or progression of the disease state. Most of the time the clinical laboratory counts white blood cells as a part of the complete blood count (CBC), performed by running

E X E R C I S E   **29**   ## PRODUCING A DIFFERENTIAL BLOOD SMEAR

SAFETY TECHNIQUE: REMEMBER TO WEAR GLOVES AND GOGGLES. PROPERLY DISPOSE OF ALL BLOODY MATERIALS.

Purpose: Practice in making blood smears produces acceptable slides.

Equipment needed: Half gross box of clean glass slides with one frosted end, **heparinized** microhematocrit glass capillary tubes, EDTA-anticoagulated blood sample, test tube rack, tube rotator, biohazard container.

Procedure:
1. Put on gloves. Some laboratories may require goggles as well.
2. Place the sample to be tested on the rotating mixer and allow it to mix for at least 3 minutes to ensure proper cell distribution.
3. Remove the sample from the mixer and carefully remove the rubber stopper from the sample, avoiding blood splashes.
4. Hold a microhematocrit capillary tube between the thumb and forefinger, inserting one end of the tube into the exposed blood sample.
5. Gentle tilt the capillary tube, allowing it to become two-thirds full with blood.
6. Place the blood tube into the test tube rack and restopper.
7. Place five glass slides on a table or other flat object.
8. Touch the capillary tube to the glass slide until a drop of blood emerges on each slide.
9. Take another glass slide and hold it between the thumb and forefinger.
10. Bring the clean slide to the slide with the drop of blood and touch the drop of blood, holding the clean slide at about a 15- to 20-degree angle. The blood should run along one side of the clean slide.
11. With a quick motion, move the clean slide away from the drop of blood, drawing the sample with it. This forms a smear. Repeat the procedure with the other slides on the table. Continue to perform this procedure until the smears you obtain have a beveled (curved) edge. After drying, the smear looks like a rainbow in the beveled area when held to reflect the room lights.
12. Properly dispose of all materials, using a hard-sided biohazardous container.

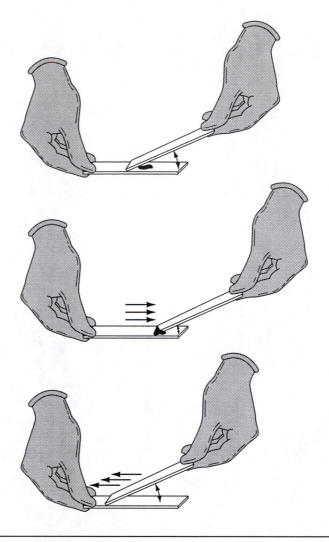

fig. 3.2. Differential slide preparation. (From Hoeltke. *Phlebotomy.* p. 113.)

a blood sample through an automated cell counter (see Unit 9 for more information on cell counters).

If the automated cell counter is not available, a laboratory scientist may have to perform a manual white blood cell count. Exercise 30 is a manual method for counting white blood cells.

TYPES OF COUNTING CHAMBERS

There are three different types of counting chambers available to the hematologist when counting manually white blood cells. The most commonly used is the **Neubauer** hemacytometer. The ruling for this hemacytometer is shown in Figure 3.3. Other **hemacytometers** are ruled using the Fuchs-Rosenthal and the Spears-Levy formula. Refer to reference textbooks for the ruling and calculations for the Fuchs-Rosenthal and Spears-Levy hemacytometers.

In the Neubauer chamber, each of the nine squares is 1 mm by 1 mm with a depth of 0.1 mm. Therefore, the results are corrected by multiplying the number of cells counted by 50 to determine the number of cells seen in 1 μl. There are two similar lined areas on the Neubauer chamber. Two different samples may be viewed to save time, or the same sample can be viewed twice to increase precision.

The following are examples of disease states that are associated with either a decrease in the WBC or an increase in the WBC. Neither list is meant to be complete. The reader should refer to reference textbooks on disease states for a more complete listing.

Some Conditions That Can Show A Decrease in the WBC

Measles	Influenza
Radiation	Cirrhosis
Infectious hepatitis	Rheumatoid arthritis
Lupus erythematosus	

Some Conditions That Can Show An Increase in the WBC

Appendicitis	Pregnancy
Abscesses	Newborns
Pneumonia	Menstruation
Tonsillitis	Ulcers
Peritonitis	Leukemia
Chickenpox	Meningitis
Erythroblastosis fetalis	Uremia

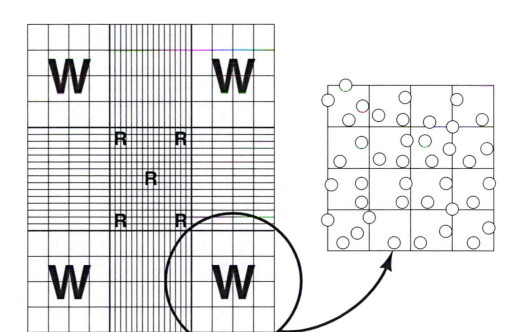

fig. 3.3. Neubauer hemacytometer. Illustration by Lora Russell.

E X E R C I S E   **30**   **MANUAL METHOD FOR COUNTING WHITE BLOOD CELLS**

SAFETY TECHNIQUE: REMEMBER TO WEAR GLOVES AND GOGGLES. PROPERLY DISPOSE OF ALL BIOHAZARDOUS MATERIALS.

Purpose: A specific amount of whole blood is diluted with acid to **lyse** red cells. Then leukocytes are counted.

Equipment Needed: Latex gloves, EDTA anticoagulated blood specimen, automatic pipettor, Thoma (WBC) pipette, hemacytometer (counting chamber), finger counter, blood mixer, diluting fluid, soft laboratory tissues or sterile gauze, and a microscope.

Procedure:

1. Place the specimen on the mixer. Mix for at least 3 minutes.
2. Note that the Thoma pipette is calibrated on the side in evenly spaced intervals, with 0.5 and 1.0 clearly marked.
3. Remove the blood tube stopper. Attach the automatic pipettor to the Thoma pipette and draw up some blood beyond the 0.5 mark.
4. Use the soft laboratory tissue to remove any blood on the outside of the pipette. Gently tap the end of the pipette. Slowly bring the blood level to EXACTLY the 0.5 mark.
5. Insert the pipette into a beaker of diluting fluid (never contaminate the stock bottle of diluting fluid). Using the automatic pipettor, draw up the diluting fluid to the **11** mark (beyond the bulge in the Thoma pipette).
6. Remove the pipette from the pipettor and place on a pipette shaker, or hold the pipette between gloved thumb and forefinger. Vigorously shake for 2 minutes.
7. Holding the pipette at an angle, allow 4 drops of brownish fluid to be expelled into a soft laboratory tissue (this represents the fluid in the pipette tip that did not mix in the bulb portion).
8. Place the special hemacytometer coverslip on the hemacytometer. Now touch the pointed end of the pipette to the edge of the coverslip. The mixed sample will now drain in between the coverslip and the counting chamber. Allow 3 to 5 minutes for the cells to settle.
9. Place the hemacytometer under the microscope. Focus using low power until a lined area with round spots on and among the lines (these are the WBC) is seen.
10. Observe the hemacytometer counting area for a good distribution of cells. Do the cells seem to be spread evenly over the entire counting area, or do they seem to be more on one side than on the other? If a good distribution is present, continue. If not, repeat the mixing process, recharge the chamber, and reobserve.

EXERCISE **30** **MANUAL METHOD FOR COUNTING WHITE BLOOD CELLS** *(continued)*

11. Count the round white cells that are found within the large "W" areas in Figure 3.3. Each of four large areas have sixteen smaller boxes in them, for a total of sixty-four. Also count any cell touching one side and the top or bottom. Most lab scientists count those touching the left side and the top, but the right and the bottom side could be used. BE CONSISTENT.

12. Using Figure 3.3, determine the number of white cells observed. Use a hand tally counter or make hash marks on a piece of paper, making one mark for each white blood cell seen.

13. The actual calculations will be performed in Exercise 31. Dispose of all hazardous materials properly. The instructor will instruct you on how to clean the hemacytometer.

NOTE: Some laboratories no longer use the Thoma pipette method. Instead, the dilution of the white blood cells is done with a Unopette®. See package insert for the Unopette® for this procedure.

EXERCISE **31** **CALCULATING A MANUAL WHITE BLOOD CELL COUNT**

Purpose: To learn to calculate a manual white blood cell count accurately.

Equipment: Paper, pencil, calculation information contained in Exercise 30.

1. The number of white blood cells seen in the diagram using the bottom and right side was 35. If the top and left side were used, the count was 37.

2. Assume that the following count was made of the four large WBC areas:
   Upper left   35
   Upper right   37
   Lower left   36
   Lower right   35
   The total for the entire area would be 143 (add the four numbers above).

3. Determine the number of white blood cells in 1 µl (microliter). Correcting for volume and dilution, using the following information:
CORRECTION FOR VOLUME Each large WBC square is 1.0 mm², with a depth of 0.1 mm for a volume of 0.1 mm³ (cubic millimeter) To calculate this, multiple 1.0 mm times 1.0 mm times 0.1 mm = 0.1 cm. Therefore, the total volume is 4 times this, or 0.4 cm. To report the result as the number of WBC/1.0 µl, correct for the volume change and use the formula **vol. cor. factor = vol. desired/vol. used**
vol. cor. factor = 1.0 µl/0.4 µl
vol. cor. factor = **2.5**

4. **CORRECTION FOR DILUTION FACTOR** The Thoma WBC Pipette was filled to the 0.5 mark with whole blood and then diluted to the 11 mark with diluting fluid, a ratio of 1:20, yielding a correction factor of **20.**

5. With the information above, calculation of the corrected WBC can be achieved. Take the total number of white cells counted (143) and multiply that number by 20 and again by 2.5, as follows:
Corrected WBC = cell count × vol. cor. factor × dil. factor
Corrected WBC = 143 × 20 × 2.5
Corrected WBC = 2860 × 2.5
Corrected WBC = 7150

6. Notice that 20 times 2.5 equals 50. It is possible to arrive at 7150 by multiplying the total number of cells observed by 50, or by dividing them by 2 and adding two zeros at the end. This moves the decimal point over two places to the right.

7. Report the results as:
WBC = 7150/µl (manual method–normal range is 5000 to 10,000/µl)

E X E R C I S E   **32**   HIGH WHITE BLOOD CELL COUNTS

Purpose: White blood counts that are above the normal range can be accurately counted by using a technique discussed below.

Procedure:

1. Students should be in small groups (three to four students) to brainstorm the following problem BEFORE READING THE SOLUTION.

2. The counting chamber has just been charged with a diluted blood sample and viewed under the microscope at 10× (low power). The field of vision looks very crowded with cells and is obviously more than a normal count. This condition may be caused by leukemia, where counts can be 100,000 or greater. ATTEMPT TO SOLVE THIS PROBLEM OF ACCURATELY COUNTING THESE CELLS.

SOLUTION TO THE PROBLEM:

To obtain a sample that is more readable, the sample must be diluted more than the usual dilution level. Obtain an RBC pipette and fill the stem to the 1.0 mark. Dilute and dilute to the 101 mark, yielding a 1 in 100 dilution. Count the four large "W" squares as usual and multiply by 250 to obtain the corrected WBC. The result is multiplied by 250 because the dilution factor correction is 100 times the volume correction factor of 2.5, which yields 250. Attempt Exercise 33, which deals with low white blood cell counts.

E X E R C I S E **33** **LOW WHITE BLOOD CELL COUNTS**

Purpose: Low white blood cell counts also pose a problem for an accurate picture for the physician to assess. A change in the diluting technique is needed to handle this problem.

Procedure:

1. Students should be in small groups (three to four students) to brainstorm the following problem BEFORE READING THE SOLUTION.
2. The counting chamber has just been charged with a diluted blood sample and viewed under the microscope at 10X (low power). The field of vision looks reduced from what is normally seen. Cancer therapy can cause a reduction in white blood cells. ATTEMPT TO SOLVE THIS PROBLEM OF ACCURATELY COUNTING THESE CELLS.

SOLUTION TO THE PROBLEM:

In this case, use a white blood cell pipette and draw the blood to the 1.0 mark (instead of the 0.5 mark). Then the diluting fluid is brought to the 11 mark. Mix and discard the first 4 drops. Count the four large areas, multiplying the result by 25. The normal dilution ratio for the WBC is 1:20. Twenty is multiplied by 2.5 (the volume correction factor), equaling 50. In this case, the dilution was only a 1:10. Ten multiplied by 2.5 is 25.

RED BLOOD CELL COUNT

Red blood cells also can be manually counted. However, today's laboratory results demand a much greater precision than can be obtained by manually counting red blood cells in a counting chamber. If the student is curious about a manual red blood cell count, a reference textbook should be referred to.

Some Conditions That Can Show An Increase in the RBC

Polycythemia vera	Moving from a high altitude to low altitude
Dehydration	Extreme physical activity

Some Conditions That Can Show A Decrease in the RBC

Any anemia	Hemorrhage
Pregnancy	Transfusion reactions
	Kidney diseases that decrease erythropoietin

THE INTERNATIONAL COMMITTEE FOR STANDARDIZATION

The International Committee for Standardization in Hematology and other international scientific committees have recommended that all units of volume be reported in liters. The conversion factor for cubic millimeters to microliters (µl) is 1 cu mm = 1.00003 µl. essentially 1 cu mm = 1 µl, which in turn equals 1×10^{-6} liters. In reporting results from WBCs, most reporting forms are in liters.

DIFFERENTIAL STAINING

When the blood counts have been completed, the next step is to perform the differential count (diff). This involves obtaining the percentage of each of the five types of leukocytes present in the blood smear. It also gives the physician information concerning morphology of the red blood cells and platelets, as well as presence of abnormal inclusion bodies and immature cell types. The differential test provides information to the physician about possible disease states. The slides must be stained as well as possible in order to obtain the important information derived from this test.

Different types of stain are used to disclose various parts of the cell. The development of hematology stains began with a Russian physician named Romanowsky. Romanowsky mixed two different stains together (one of acid nature and one of basic nature) and attempted to stain blood smears. These stains are now normally called polychrome stains because of the different colors found in the cells.

E X E R C I S E   **TRANSPOSING cu mm READINGS TO MICROLITERS**

Purpose: To demonstrate reporting results in liters.

Equipment Needed: Results from Exercise 33.

Procedure:
1. Obtain the results obtained for the manual white blood cell counts in Exercise 31.
2. Calculate results using liters:

Modifications of Romanowsky's formula have yielded Wright's stain, an alcohol solution with the combined eosin (acid) and methylene blue (basic) dyes. This stain allows the hematologist a broad range of colors to stain the internal parts of the white cells. A buffer solution is used with this stain because of the acidity of the water used in the procedure. Another modification is the Giemsa stain. A modified Wright's stain called the *Quick Stain* does not use a buffer because the procedure is so fast. Exercises 35 and 36 illustrate staining techniques used often in the hematology laboratory.

SPECIAL STAINING PROCEDURES

BONE MARROW STAINS

The pathologist is generally involved with performing bone marrow examinations. However, bone marrow examinations are an excellent way to become familiar with immature cells, which may be seen in pathologic differential smears.

STAINING CELLULAR ORGANELLES

Some pathologists require that certain cellular components be stained for, because these organelles can be characteristic of a particular disease state. Clinical laboratory scientists usually have some background in staining techniques and in various stains used to view these organelles. Such techniques include:

- Use of Wright's or Quick stain to detect a distinguishable nucleus.
- Use of Periodic Acid-Shiff Reaction/Stain to identify and classify immature cells of the bone marrow and blood.
- Acid phosphatase stain used to identify hair cell leukemia.
- Heinz body staining (bodies appearing in red blood cells due to injury or exposure to a specific drug) by use of brilliant cresyl blue or a methyl violet solution.
- Myeloperoxidase stain to differentiate immature myeloid and lymphocytic cells. Immature myeloid cells stain with myeloperoxidase stain.
- Alkaline phosphatase staining to aid in identifying certain white blood cells, including neutrophils, band cells, and metamyelocytes.
- Perodixase staining, where certain white cells with granules will stain, while nongranulated cells will not stain; useful in helping to identify a leukemia cell type.
- Esterase staining, where specific esterase stains granulocytic blast forms and nonspecific esterase stains monocytic blasts.

E X E R C I S E **DIFFERENTIAL STAINING WITH WRIGHT'S STAIN**

SAFETY TECHNIQUE: WEAR GLOVES.

Purpose: Differential staining with Wright's Stain allows the hematologist to see specific characteristics of white blood cells.

Equipment Needed: Differential smears, Wright's stain (in powder form or made up), staining racks, timer, buffer solution, drying area, biohazard container

Procedure:

1. Place the slides to be stained on a staining rack in a sink. Stain can splash off the slide when the buffer is applied.
2. Make sure the smeared side of the slide is facing up.
3. Apply Wright's stain evenly over the entire slide. (If your instructor does not have Wright's stain already made up, a reference textbook may have to be consulted for preparing the stain and buffer. This exercise assumes that the Wright's stain is already made up. Most laboratories buy prepared stains since time does not allow for preparation of stains.)
4. Time this staining procedure with the timer for 3 minutes (this time can be adjusted upward or downward, depending on the results of the staining).
5. Add the buffer solution.
6. Set the timer for 5 minutes and then wash off the stain/buffer mixture with distilled water.
7. Holding the slide in one hand, take a soft laboratory tissue and wipe only a small section of the underside of the slide. If no cells are removed with this first wipe proceed to wipe off the entire underside of the slide. If cells are removed with the first wipe turn the slide over and try again.
8. Allow the slide to drain off excess water by standing it on end touching a paper towel or soft laboratory tissue and allow to air dry.
9. Once the slide is dry, it is ready to be viewed under the microscope, starting with low power. When in focus, turn the objective slightly toward the OIL lens and add a drop of oil to the slide. Snap the lens in place to view the cells individually. Readjustment of the objective should not be necessary, but fine adjustment may be needed.
10. Are the cells stained properly? Are you able to see clear differences? Consult your instructor.
11. Dispose of all biohazardous materials properly.

EXERCISE **36** BONE MARROW EXAMINATION

SAFETY TECHNIQUE: WEAR GLOVES.

Purpose: The examination of the bone marrow can provide invaluable information about the health of the patient.

Equipment Needed: Six to eight clean glass slides for making smears, various stains, and jar of preservative for cell block. (If fresh bone marrow is not available, students will observe bone marrow slides provided by the instructor.)

Procedure:
1. The sample is drawn from the iliac crest or more rarely from the sternum. This procedure is performed by a pathologist, usually aided by a clinical laboratory scientist who makes the smears and preserves the cell block. There is some pain involved in the bone marrow tap.
2. Have six to eight slides prepared to smear and a small container with preservative in it.
3. Place a larger sample (the cell block) into the preservative.
4. Smear the slides and allow to dry while returning to the laboratory.
5. Stain them with Wright's stain or other special stains as requested by the pathologist.

EXERCISE **37** ESTERASE STAINING OF LEUKOCYTES

SAFETY TECHNIQUE: WEAR GLOVES.

Principle: Esterases are enzymes that act on specific substrates. The specific esterases stain granulocytic blasts, and the nonspecific esterases stain monocytic blast forms. This exercise will use the nonspecific esterase stain.

Equipment needed: Sigma Diagnostic Kit Numbers 386-1 and 90-A1, deionized water, ACS-grade acetone, absolute methanol, glass slides, EDTA, or heparinized blood sample.

Procedure:
1. Follow all procedures as to development of reagents as described in kits.

E X E R C I S E **37** **ESTERASE STAINING OF LEUKOCYTES**
(continued)

2. Mix nine parts deionized water to one part citrate solution. Stable for 1 week.
3. Mix 19 ml of dilute citrate solution with 27 ml of acetone and 5 ml methanol. Stable for 8 hours in a tightly capped bottle.
4. Fix prepared slides for 30 seconds in above solution, rinse in deionized water, and air dry.
5. To 50 ml of Trizma 7.6 dilute buffer (made by adding one part concentrated buffer with nine parts deionized water), add one capsule of fast blue RR salt. Make sure Trizma has been prewarmed to 37°C. When salt is dissolved, add 2 ml of alpha-naphthyl acetate solution and mix for 30 seconds. Add resulting solution to staining tray.
6. Place slides in staining tray for 30 minutes and cover with brown or opaque cover to protect from light. Wash slides in running water for 3 minutes. Stained slides can be counterstained with hematoxylin stain for 5 minutes and washed in tap water.
7. Air dry slide and use coverslip with mounting medium to seal slide.
8. Examine for black granulation in monocytes. Neutrophils lack granulation, but lymphocytes may show a very light, speckled staining pattern.
9. Dispose of all biohazardous materials in a puncture-proof biohazard container.

SUMMARY

One of the most commonly ordered laboratory tests is the complete blood count (CBC). This test consists of a white blood cell count (WBC), a red blood cell count (RBC), a hemoglobin level (Hb or Hgb), a hematocrit (Hct), red blood cell indices (MCV, MCH, MCHC), a platelet count (on modern cell counters), and a differential. These tests can be performed on an automated cell counter using EDTA-anticoagulated blood.

Differential testing involves the identification of 100 white blood cells on a stained blood smear and determining their percentages. Additional information such as morphology of blood cells and platelets can also be determined, as well as the presence of abnormal cells and inclusion bodies. Although these tests are performed on automated equipment, laboratory scientists often have to perform a manual differential count when abnormalities are suspected. A differential blood smear is stained with Wright's stain. Much practice is necessary to learn to make a readable smear.

When a manual white count is necessary (if automated equipment fails), the student performs this count using a counting chamber. The Neubauer hemacytometer is the most commonly used counting chamber. Results must be obtained by correcting for the volume of the chamber and the correction for the dilution factor. Special techniques are used to count high and low white blood counts manually.

Red blood cells should not be counted manually. Results are too inaccurate due to the high volume of red blood cells in a sample.

The International Committee for Standardization has recommended that all units of volume be reported in liters. The student should be familiar with conversions of cubic millimeters to microliters.

Staining the differential smear requires careful technique. The Wright's stain is used for differential staining, allowing the hematologist to see specific characteristics of white blood cells.

Other special staining procedures that may be encountered in the hematology department include bone marrow stains and other specific stains that highlight certain cellular components, which may be characteristic of a particular disease state.

REVIEW QUESTIONS

1. What is the dilution factor when using a Thoma WBC pipette?
   a. 1:10
   b. 1:20
   c. 1:200
   d. 1:100
2. When staining with Wright's stain, it may be necessary to use a
   _____ to obtain acceptable slides.
   a. buffer
   b. counter stain
   c. long staining period
   d. short staining period
3. Red blood cells are not usually counted manually in the clinical laboratory because
   a. physicians never order red blood cell counts
   b. the red blood cell count is not important
   c. the manual red blood cell count is not accurate due to the vast numbers of cells
   d. none of the above
4. The depth of the area encountered on the hemacytometer for counting cells is
   a. 0.04 mm
   b. 1.0 mm
   c. 0.1 mm
   d. 4.0 mm

5. In making the calculations for a white blood cell count, the combination of dilution correction factor times the volume correction factor yields a factor of
   a. 10
   b. 20
   c. 40
   d. 50

6. How many large squares must be counted to obtain a white blood cell count?
   a. 5
   b. 4
   c. 2
   d. 1

7. Which of the following are peroxidase positive?
   a. myeloblasts
   b. lymphoblasts
   c. lymphocytes
   d. monocytes

8. The acid phosphatase staining technique is used primarily for the identification of
   a. hairy cell leukemia
   b. acute myelogenous leukemia
   c. chronic myelogenous leukemia
   d. reticulocytes

9. Esterase staining
   a. helps differentiate red blood cells and white blood cells
   b. is used to stain platelets
   c. is used to differentiate granulocytic blasts and monocytic blast forms
   d. can substitute for Wright's stain when preparing differential slides

10. When performing a differential, the best place to read the stained smear is
    a. the feathered edge
    b. the area where the cells are most numerous
    c. the area where cells are far apart
    d. directly in the middle of the slide

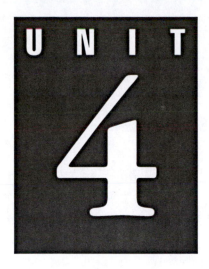

White Blood Cells (Leukocytes)

GLOSSARY

agranulocytes historical term pertaining to lymphocytes, monocytes, and megakaryocytes.

antigen any protein or carbohydrate that causes a lymphocyte to produce antibodies.

Auer rods red staining rods that can appear in myeloblast cells; can indicate acute myeloblastic leukemia.

azurophilic granules small inclusions in the cytoplasm of cells that stain sky blue.

basophil least prevalent white blood cell; may play a role in acute allergic reactions.

blood islets groups of cells found in the yolk sac that develop into the blood vessels and blood cells.

eosinophil white blood cell active in allergic reactions and parasitic infections.

extravascular originating outside of the blood vessels.

gestation development of the embryo from a fertilized egg.

granulocytes cells with a segmented nucleus and dense, clumped chromatin.

hemocytoblast cell that is believed to be the origin of all other types of white blood cells.

hepatic phase second phase of blood cell development; confined to the liver beginning at week 6 of intrauterine life.

intrauterine time spent within the uterus.

leukemia malignant (cancerous) disorder of the blood-forming tissues, mainly the bone marrow, lymph nodes, and spleen; often presents as an abnormal increase in the white blood cell count.

lymphocytes white blood cells primarily involved in cellular and antibody immunity.

megakaryocytes large cells that break apart in the bone marrow to form platelets.

megaloblastic phase first stage of blood cell development starting within the yolk sac in the first month of life.

mesoderm middle layer of embryonic cells forming the granulocytes.

myeloid phase last stage of blood cell development taking place in the bone marrow; starts in the fifth month of fetal development.

mitosis normal cell division producing two identical cells.

monocytes largest white blood cells involved in phagocytosis.

neutrophil most prominent white blood cell with a three or four lobed nucleus.

pernicious anemia disease affecting the red blood cells, causing a decrease in oxygen-carrying capacity.

phagocytic method of cell eating in which false feet encircle the article to be consumed.

Philadelphia chromosome (Ph[1]) balanced translocation between long arms of chromosome 9 and 22 seen in erythroid, granulocytic, monocytic, and megakaryocytic cells; found in 90% of cases of chronic myelogenous leukemia.

platelets also called thrombocytes; cell fragments that aid in blood clotting.

stem cell undifferentiated mononuclear cell having the potential to differentiate into one or more cell lines.

thrombocytes another term for platelets.

INTRODUCTION

Unlike the red blood cell, there is more than one type of white blood cell (leukocyte) circulating at any one time. The functions of leukocytes are diverse and numerous. In contrast to red blood cells (erythrocytes), white blood cells primarily function outside blood vessels. They can cross membranes better than red blood cells. Changes in either function or number of leukocytes reflect a definite change in the body's function, providing valuable diagnostic information to the physician.

ORIGIN OF BLOOD CELLS

Blood cells have their origin in the **blood islets** found within the yolk sac of the developing human embryo in the womb. Blood islets are groups of cells that, through the process of cell **mitosis**, cause cells to extend toward each other to form tubes. The central portion of the cell mass becomes the first blood cells, or else it breaks apart, releasing cytoplasm to form the first plasma. If the mother's immune system is functioning properly, her antibodies will protect her infant, and so the immediate need for white cells is minimal. The first cells within the embryo are red blood cells to carry oxygen to the developing embryo.

White blood cells may arise as early as the third day of **gestation**, but usually arise during the first 2 months in the **megaloblastic phase** in the yolk sac's blood islets. The **hepatic phase** begins in the liver from about 6 to 9 weeks of life, aided by the spleen and thymus until about the fifth month. The granular leukocytes have their origin **extravascularly** from the **mesoderm**, but migrate through the capillary walls and become established in the blood vessels. The last phase is the **myeloid phase**, beginning in the fifth **intrauterine** month and finally being established within the bone marrow spaces. In times of need the spleen, liver, and kidneys can become cell producers.

CELL LINE ORIGINS

Each cell line has its origin in a **stem cell**, an undifferentiated mononuclear cell having the potential to differentiate into one or more cell lines. Some authors refer to this cell as the **hemocytoblast**. The fact that the **Philadelphia chromosome (Ph[1])** is found in patients with chronic myelogenous **leukemia** (CML), in immature erythrocytes, megakaryocytes, monocytes, neutrophils, basophils, and eosinophils indicates that these cells have a single origin. The Philadelphia chromosome is not found in lymphocytes, however.

Most of what has been learned about the stem cell and its role in the formation of the various cell lines comes from removal of generalized bone marrow, growing the cells in culture, and observing for the formation of cell lines. See Table 4.1 for a review of cellular development.

MYELOID CELL LINE

The myeloid cell line forms the red blood cells, the granulocytes (neutrophils, eosinophils, and basophils), the monocytes, and the megakaryocytes. Red blood

Table 4.1.

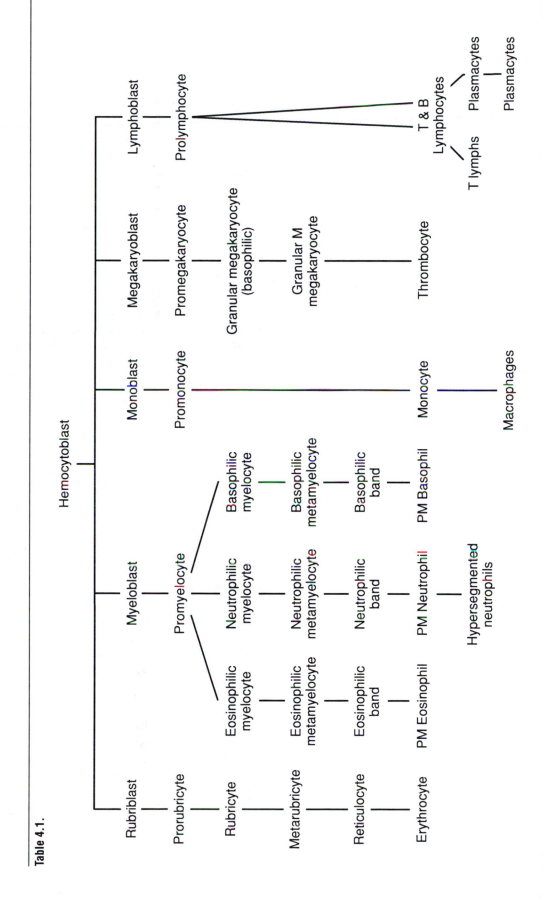

cell maturation will be dealt with in Unit 6, and megakaryocytes will be discussed in Unit 8.

Granulocytes vs. Agranulocytes

The **granulocytes** have a segmented nucleus with dense, clumped chromatin. The cytoplasm contains specific granules, being fine and staining violet-pink in the **neutrophil**, appearing large and bright orange-red in the **eosinophil**, appearing large and purplish-black in the **basophil**. The neutrophils usually have a three- or four-segmented nucleus, whereas the eosinophils and basophils have a bilobed nucleus (if it can be seen through the large amount of granules). The three granulocytic leukocytes are illustrated in Figure 4.1.

Agranulocytes is a historical term used to describe the **lymphocytes**, **monocytes**, and **megakaryocytes**. They are called agranular because their granules are not as evident by normal light microscope techniques but may show up using the electron microscope. Lymphocytes are the second most common cell found within the differential cell count. Monocytes are approximately 2% to 9% in the count.

Megakaryocytes are the largest cells in the hematopoietic tissue. They are normally seen only in the bone marrow. However, if a compound fracture of a bone occurs, they may be seen for a short period of time in the peripheral circulation. These cells produce the **platelets** (also called **thrombocytes**), fragments of cells pinched off from the megakaryocytes. Cells resembling large lymphocytes with small attached platelets have been identified as micromegakaryocytes. They are sometimes seen in chronic myelogenous leukemia.

THE GRANULOCYTES

The granulocytes are the most common white blood cell in circulation and will constitute the major portion of this unit. They are characterized by the presence of granules in their cytoplasm, including those that accept acid stain, those that accept basic stain, and those that are neutral in their staining characteristics.

The first cell in the granulocytic (also called myelocytic) line is the myeloblast, followed in successively mature stages by the promyelocyte, myelocyte, metamyelocyte, band cell, and adult segmented cell.

THE MYELOBLAST

The myeloblast is the first committed cell in the granulocytic series. It is distinguished by the dark blue staining cytoplasm, the presence of nucleoli, a homogenous nuclear pattern, and a large nuclear/cytoplasm ratio of about 6:1. There are usually two oval or circular shaped areas inside of the nucleus associated with protein synthesis. These are called nucleoli. There can be more than two nucleoli. The nucleolus stains pale blue, indicating the presence of RNA. This cell, like most blast forms, is a large cell, being about 10 to 18 μm in diameter. The myeloblast may have **Auer rods** (Auer bodies) in the cytoplasm in acute myeloblastic leukemias. These red-staining rods can also be found in monocytes.

One technique of identifying myeloblasts or other blast cells is to "look for the company they keep"—observing what cells are found around them. If the cells in the general vicinity are of the granulocytic series, then it is reasonable that the blast cell might be a myeloblast.

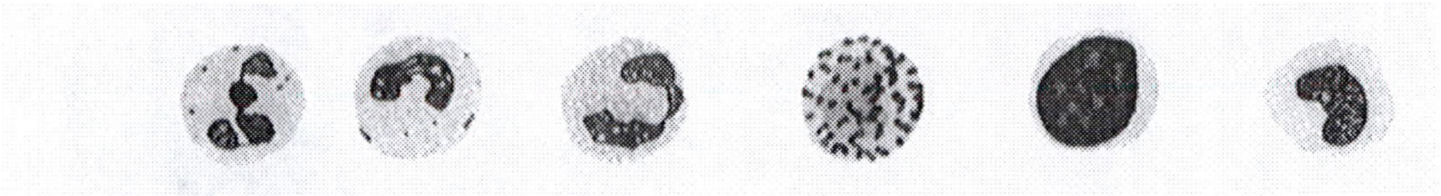

	Segmented Neutrophil	Netrophilic Band (Stab)	Eosinophil	Basophil	Lymphocyte	Monocyte
Cell Size (μm)	10–15	10–15	10–15	10–15	8–15	12–20
Nucleus						
shape	2–5 lobes	sausage or U-shaped	bilobed	segmented	round, oval	horseshoe
structure	coarse	coarse	coarse	difficult to see	smudged (smoothly stained)	folded, convoluted
Cytoplasm						
amount	abundant	abundant	abundant	abundant	scant	abundant
color	pink-tan	pink-tan	pink-tan	pink-tan	clear blue	opaque, blue-gray
inclusions	small, lilac granules	small, lilac granules	coarse, orange-red granules	coarse, blue-black granules	occasional red-purple granules	ground-glass appearance

fig. 4.1. Leukocyte identification scheme. (From Marshall. *Fundamental Skills for the Clinical Laboratory Professional.* p. 360.)

E X E R C I S E **38** **IDENTIFICATION OF GRANULOCYTIC CELLS**

Purpose: The hematologist must be proficient in the accurate identification of various white blood cells.

Equipment Needed: Blood smears provided by the instructor or student-made smears.

Procedure:
1. Using the low power objective, focus on the smear.
2. Place a drop of oil on the smear and swing the oil immersion lens (100×) in place. Refocus if necessary.
3. Locate the thin (feathered) area of the smear.
4. Using the mechanical stage apparatus, move the smear upward, then to the left, then down, observing for granulocytes, as shown in Figure 4.1. At this stage, the student will benefit from having available color reference charts that show the different white blood cells.
5. Locate a neutrophil, eosinophil, and basophil. Make a drawing of these cells.

THE PROMYELOCYTE

The second cell in the series, still capable of dividing and producing a total of four myelocytes (two from each daughter cell of the myeloblast), is the promyelocyte. It is slightly larger than the myeloblast, being about 12 to 20 μm in diameter and showing an oval nucleus with slightly clumped chromatin. The nucleus

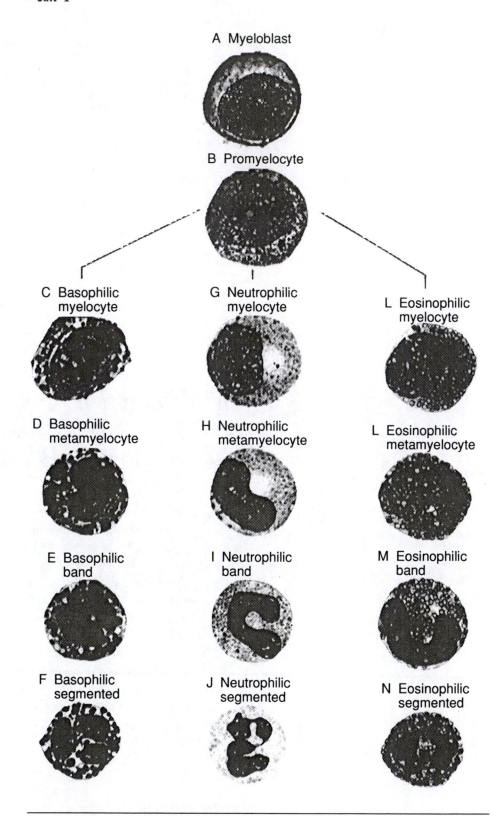

A Myeloblast

B Promyelocyte

C Basophilic
myelocyte

G Neutrophilic
myelocyte

L Eosinophilic
myelocyte

D Basophilic
metamyelocyte

H Neutrophilic
metamyelocyte

L Eosinophilic
metamyelocyte

E Basophilic
band

I Neutrophilic
band

M Eosinophilic
band

F Basophilic
segmented

J Neutrophilic
segmented

N Eosinophilic
segmented

fig. 4.2. Development of the myeloid series. (From Marshall. *Fundamental Skills for the Clinical Laboratory Professional.* p. 311.)

has two or more nucleoli, but they may be less distinct, staining light blue. The cytoplasm is still staining bluish to purple with a few large primary granules dark blue in color. The nucleus/cytoplasm ratio is now 4:1. In the normal bone marrow, this cell is usually associated with the blast forms.

THE MYELOCYTE

The myelocyte is the third stage of maturation in the granulocytic series. This cell is the last cell to reproduce in the series, yielding a total of eight daughter cells (two from each of the four promyelocytes). There are three types of myelocytes: the most common is the neutrophil, but eosinophils and basophils also develop from an immature myelocyte during maturation.

The myelocyte is the same size as the blast, that is, 12 to 18 μm in diameter. There is a nucleus/cytoplasmic ratio of 2:1, indicating that the nucleus is clumping down on itself. This yields the appearance of more cytoplasm. Nucleoli are absent and the nucleus is round or oval, with light purple clumped chromatin.

Origin of Secondary Granules

Secondary granules arise at the myelocytic stage. Some granules accept eosin, an acid stain. The cell may be red to orange in color, depending on the age of the stain (the redder the granule, the fresher the stain). These cells will become eosinophils. Some accept a basic stain called methylene blue stain, dark bluish to purple in color. These cells will become basophils. The third group of cells will stain with light purple granules and will become neutrophils.

THE METAMYELOCYTE

The metamyelocyte is a very specialized cell. It is the first cell that is easily identified by the shape of the nucleus (see Figure 4.2). The nucleus is distinctly indented to produce a kidney bean shape. The nucleus is composed of dense clumped chromatin and stains dark purple in color. The cytoplasm is abundant and pink, with the nucleus/cytoplasmic ratio being 1.5:1.0. The cell is about 10 to 18 μm. The terms *neutrophilic, basophilic,* and *eosinophilic* must accompany the term metamyelocyte, depending on the stained granules present.

THE BAND

This cell (also called *stab*) is normally found in the peripheral circulation in very low amounts (0% to 5%). The band is distinguished by its nuclear shape of a rubber band, curved in the form of a thin sausage. The chromatin of the nucleus is very condensed and dark purple when stained with Wright's stain. The nucleus/cytoplasmic ratio is 1:2, yielding a cell with what appears to be more cytoplasm. The secondary granules sometimes obscure the nucleus of the basophil and the eosinophil, but the nucleus of the neutrophil is usually evident. These cells show an increase in infectious states and will mature in the circulation. Physicians are often interested in the band count as a way of determining if a patient has an infection.

The distinction between band stage and the fully mature neutrophil stage is that the nucleus is not segmented in any way. There may be an indentation of the nucleus, but the two sides do not meet.

EXERCISE **39** **IDENTIFICATION OF THE MYELOID SERIES**

Purpose: Proper identification of the myeloid series is critical in accessing various disease states, especially in leukemia identification and treatment.

Equipment Needed: Blood smears provided by the instructor (bone marrow slides will show normal development, leukemia slides will show malignant development).

Procedure:

1. Using the oil immersion lens (100×), bring the smear into focus.
2. Locate an area associated with myeloid maturation.
3. Locate various immature forms (myeloblast, promyelocyte, myelocyte, metamyelocyte). Have your instructor check your identifications. A reference chart is indispensable for identification of these forms. (Also see Figure 4.2.)
4. Repetition in this exercise is very important. Before you complete the exercise, you should have an idea of the differences in each of the immature stages.

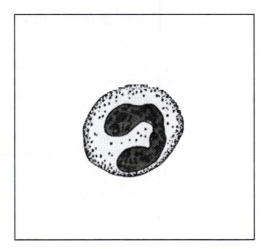

fig. 4.3. The band cell. (From Marshall. *Fundamental Skills for the Clinical Laboratory Professional.* p. 316.)

THE NEUTROPHIL

The neutrophil has several names, including the *polymorphonuclear granulocyte, PMN, seg,* and *poly.* It is the most common and most mature cell in the granulocytic series. The cell is segmented, often having three segmented portions of the nucleus. The longer it remains in circulation, the more segments it produces. When the number of segments seen is six or more, it is called a hypersegmented

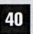

E X E R C I S E 40 IDENTIFICATION OF BAND CELLS

Purpose: Band cells are the first cell of the myeloid series normally seen in the peripheral blood smear, indicating the presence of infection if seen in increased amounts.

Equipment Needed: Bone marrow smears or normal blood smears provided by your instructor, or student-made smears.

Procedure:
1. Using the oil immersion lens (100×), bring the blood smear into focus.
2. Locate the thin area of the smear.
3. Locate several bands and make a drawing of the cells.

neutrophil. Excessive segments can be an indication of **pernicious anemia** and can also be a hereditary anomaly.

The nucleus/cytoplasmic ratio is 1:3. In most cases, the granules in the neutrophil are difficult to see because of their small size. The entire cell size is 10 to 15 μm. This cell is the first line of defense against invasion from bacteria. It is **phagocytic** and consumes both bacteria and worn out body cells. This cell makes up 50% to 70% of the normal differential count.

THE EOSINOPHIL

The eosinophil is distinguished from the neutrophil by the presence of reddish-orange granules in the cytoplasm and a bilobed nucleus instead of a trilobed one. It functions to suppress inflammation in the body tissues. Eosinophils have a diurnal habit, that is, their numbers increase or decrease on a daily basis in a predictable manner. They are found to increase in allergic reactions and in para-

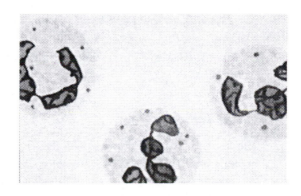

fig. 4.4. The neutrophil. (From Marshall. *Fundamental Skills for the Clinical Laboratory Professional.* Centerpiece, #1.)

EXERCISE 41 IDENTIFICATION OF NEUTROPHILS

SAFETY TECHNIQUE: WEAR GLOVES.

Purpose: The neutrophil is the most common cell in the peripheral blood smear.

Equipment Needed: Blood smears provided by the instructor (preferably the same smears used in Exercise 40).

Procedure:
1. Using the oil immersion lens (100×), bring the smear into focus.
2. Locate the thin area of the smear.
3. Locate a neutrophil and make a drawing of it.
4. Locate a band cell and have your instructor verify that you can see the difference between the neutrophil and the band. Draw a band and compare the drawing to your neutrophil drawing.

sitic infections. The normal value of these cells is 2 to 4 out of 100. The coloration of the granules is governed by the age of the stain used; if the stain is older, the granules will be more orange. An eosinophil is seen in Figure 4.1. Consult a hematology reference textbook with color plates to visualize the color of this cell after being stained with Wright's stain.

The total eosinophil count is performed to aid the physician in the diagnosis and treatment of allergic infections and infestations with worms and other large parasites. The total eosinophil count involves diluting EDTA blood with a fluid that causes lysis of the red blood cells and stains the eosinophils.

Some Conditions That Can Show Eosinopenia (Decreased Eosinophils)

Cushing's disease	After major surgery
Severe infections	Shock

Some Conditions That Can Show Eosinophilia (Increased Eosinophils):

Allergies	Skin diseases
Hodgkin's disease	Parasitic infections
Tuberculosis	Chronic myelogenous leukemia

THE BASOPHIL

The basophilic granulocyte, like the eosinophil, has a bilobed nucleus. The nucleus can be covered by granules that may obscure it. It is the least common and smallest granulocytic cell in the peripheral circulation, having a normal value of 0.5% to 1%.

The basophil has a nucleus/cytoplasm ratio of 1:1 and averages 10 to 15 μm in diameter. This cell contains large amounts of histamine and heparin. It is some-

EXERCISE **42** THE TOTAL EOSINOPHIL COUNT

SAFETY TECHNIQUE: WEAR GLOVES.

Purpose: The eosinophil count is used to determine if eosinophils are increased in the circulation. A significant increase in this population can provide the physician with valuable information. Some disorders do show a decrease in total eosinophils as well.

Equipment Needed: Unopette® system, EDTA blood, hemacytometer, hand tally counter for cells, soft laboratory tissues, microscope, biohazard disposal unit, gloves.

Procedure:
1. Thoroughly read the directions for using the Unopette® system.
2. Using the cap of the Unopette® system, puncture the diaphragm of the reservoir that is placed on a hard surface.
3. Fill the capillary pipette of the cap with EDTA anticoagulated blood by touching the blood with the pipet held at a slight angle to the specimen.
4. Wipe off any excess blood from the outside of the pipet with a soft laboratory tissue.
5. Gently squeeze the reservoir between the index finger and thumb. Insert the capillary pipette into the diluent/stain in the reservoir.
6. Release the reservoir. The blood sample will be drawn into the diluent/stain.
7. Rinse the pipette by *gently* squeezing the reservoir and releasing it several times. The diluent will enter the pipette and be drawn back into the reservoir.
8. Leave the pipette in the diluent. Place an index finger (gloved) over the top of the pipette and the thumb on the opposite side. Mix by inversion.
9. Allow to stand for 5 minutes. Charge the Neubauer counting chamber with the stained cells. Be sure to discard the first four drops. The stain will be picked up by the eosinophils in the sample.
10. Place a moistened piece of filter paper into the top of a Petri dish. Place the charged hemocytometer inside the dish for 10 minutes to allow the cells to settle.
11. Using the hand tally and a microscope that is set to low power objective, count the number of eosinophils seen on both sides of the counting chamber.
12. Calculation with the Neubauer counting chamber:
    Let us say that the total count was 40. The eosinophil count would be:

| Total number of eosinophils counted | × dilution correction factor | × volume correction factor |

E X E R C I S E **42** THE TOTAL EOSINOPHIL COUNT *(continued)*

The dilution correction factor is 10; the volume correction factor is calculated by multiplying the 9 mm² of the ruled area times the depth of the counting chamber (0.1 mm deep). Since you counted two sides, you would multiply 9 × 0.1 × 2 to equal 1.8 cu mm.

40 eos × 10 dilution factor ÷ by 1.8

The result is $\frac{400}{1.8}$ = 222 eosinophils per cubic millimeter.

Normal values: 50 to 400 eosinophils per cu mm

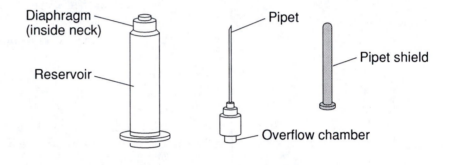

fig. 4.5. The Unopette system. (From Hoeltke. *Phlebotomy.* Delmar, p. 84.)

times associated with bleeding disorders because of the heparin, and with vasoconstriction and bronchoconstriction because of the histamine. There also is some indication that basophils are associated with allergic reactions when their numbers show a definite increase. They last only a short time in the peripheral circulation.

THE LYMPHOCYTIC SERIES

The lymphocytic series of cells, categorized as agranulocytes, are involved with the immune system and its response to invading organisms. The series consists of several types of cells, including the T-lymphocyte (of which there are several subgroups), the B-lymphocyte, the plasma cell (which is an activated B-lymphocyte found in lymph nodes), natural killer cells (NK), and non-B, non-T cells. The origin of these cells has been debated for many years, but they are now considered to arise from the pluripotential stem cell as are all other groups. Two types of lymphoid organs are associated with these cells: the primary lymphoid organs, such as the bone marrow and thymus, and the secondary lymphoid organs, such as the gut-associated lymphoid tissue (GALT), lymph nodes, and spleen.

EXERCISE **43** # IDENTIFICATION OF EOSINOPHILS AND BASOPHILS

Purpose: Eosinophils are distinguished by their red/orange granules, whereas basophils are identified by their purplish-black granules.

Equipment Needed: Blood smears provided by the instructor.

Procedure:
1. Using the oil immersion lens (100×), bring the smear into focus.
2. Locate the thin area of the smear.
3. Locate an eosinophil and make a drawing of the cell.
4. Locate a basophil and make a drawing of it as well. Compare the two cells.

THE LYMPHOBLAST

The lymphoblast is the most immature cell in the lymphocytic series, present normally in the bone marrow. The cell is part of the mitotic pool and therefore goes through normal mitosis to produce many copies of itself. Its identification is difficult because, like other blast forms, it has the general characteristics of a blast form.

The lymphoblast is a large cell, 10 to 20 μm in diameter with a nucleus/cytoplasmic ratio of 5:1. The cytoplasm forms an irregular outline with blue color to it, particularly along the outer edge. The nucleus is usually eccentric and can be either round or oval. The nuclear chromatin is dark purple with two nucleoli staining light blue found within it.

The identifying characteristics include the irregular cytoplasm border, light staining areas around the nucleus (perinuclear area), and dark staining cytoplasm on the periphery. The student can refer to hematology reference textbooks with color plates to see the color of this cell. When leukemic lymphoblasts are seen in the peripheral blood, their presence can indicate an acute lymphocytic leukemia (Figure 4.6).

THE PROLYMPHOCYTE

The prolymphocyte is a cell that is not morphologically mature, residing normally in the bone marrow. This cell is more mature than the lymphoblast. The prolymphocyte is often identified by immunological tests because morphological observations are not always accurate in classifying these in-between cells.

The characteristics of the prolymphocyte are essentially the same as the blast form, but with less distinction of the nucleoli and a less basophilic (blue coloration) cytoplasm. Again, the student should refer to a hematology reference textbook to study the morphology of this cell.

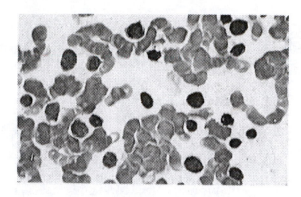

fig. 4.6. Acute lymphocytic leukemia. (From Marshall. *Fundamental Skills for the Clinical Laboratory Professional.* p. 329.)

THE LYMPHOCYTE

The lymphocyte is the second most common cell in peripheral circulation, representing from 20% to 30% of the average differential count (refer to Figure 4.1 for normal lymph morphology). These cells are associated with the immune system developing both cellular and humoral responses to invasion from foreign (and sometimes one's own) proteins.

Lymphocytes are the smallest nucleated cell in the peripheral circulation. For the most part, lymphocytes in the peripheral circulation are found in two forms. There are young lymphocytes with clear cytoplasm and a dark staining round nucleus. There are also mature lymphs, with only a very dark staining dense nucleus and no cytoplasm. Lymphs are just slightly larger than red blood cells at 7 to 10 μ in diameter, with the nucleus making up about 90% of the cell size. Some azurophilic granules may be evident. These granules are different from those of the myelocytic series, in that they do not pick up peroxidase stain and are negative for this stain.

Lymphocytes are cells that respond to antigenic stimulation. Those lymphs associated with cellular immunity are called T-lymphs and those associated with humoral immunity are called B-lymphs. The B-lymphs change to become antibody-producing cells called plasma cells upon stimulation and activation (Figure 4.7).

Atypical Lymphocytes

Lymphocytes can have an altered appearance during particular disease states. The cytoplasm of these cells tends to become more intensely blue in color. This lymph can also show increases or decreases in cytoplasmic volume. Cells with increased cytoplasmic volume, when stained with Wright's stain, tend to show indentations by adjacent structures, especially red blood cells. The cytoplasm can appear to be flowing around and almost engulfing such structures. The cells also tend to have an increased number of nonspecific azurophilic granules in the cytoplasm. Nuclear changes can also be apparent, such as changing shape to become oval or kidney-shaped, with the nucleus becoming looser and more delicate. These lymphocytes are called *atypical* (also reactive) and are actually stimulated T-lymphs (Figure 4.8). They are seen in mumps, viral pneumonia, infectious hepatitis, infectious mononucleosis, cytomegalovirus, and toxoplasmosis.

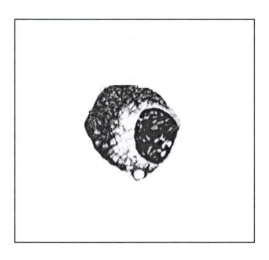

fig. 4.7. The plasma cell. (From Marshall. *Fundamental Skills for the Clinical Laboratory Professional.* p. 316.)

E X E R C I S E   **IDENTIFICATION OF LYMPHOCYTES**

SAFETY FEATURE: WEAR GLOVES.

Purpose: Lymphocytes are the second most numerous cell in peripheral circulation.

Equipment Needed: Blood smears provided by the instructor or student-made smears.

Procedure:
1. Using the oil immersion lens (100×), bring the smear into focus.
2. Locate the thin area of the smear.
3. Locate a lymphocyte and make a drawing of that cell. Include in the drawing lymphs with cytoplasm and lymphs with little if any cytoplasm.

Optional Exercise: Students prepare a report on the role of lymphocytes in HIV infection.

Infectious mononucleosis, also called *IM*, is caused by the presence of the Epstein-Barr virus. When the laboratory scientist sees many atypical lymphocytes in the differential smear, infectious mononucleosis is often suspected. A specific agglutination test, the Monospot® test, can be used to verify the virus.

Sometimes patients with all the clinical manifestations and peripheral blood findings of IM may not be positive. This can indicate the presence of a different viral infection, such as cytomegalovirus.

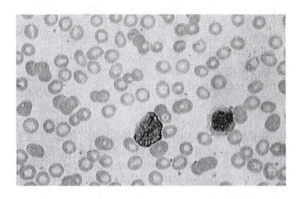

fig. 4.8. The atypical lymphocyte. (From Marshall. *Fundamental Skills for the Clinical Laboratory Professional.* p. 327.)

E X E R C I S E 45 IDENTIFICATION OF ATYPICAL LYMPHOCYTES

SAFETY TECHNIQUE: WEAR GLOVES.

Purpose: Atypical lymphocytes can appear in the peripheral circulation when a patient has an acute viral infection, most commonly associated with infectious mononucleosis.

Equipment Needed: Blood smears provided by the instructor.

Procedure:
1. Using the oil immersion lens (100×), bring the smear into focus.
2. Locate the thin area of the smear.
3. Locate an atypical lymphocyte and make a drawing of that cell. Compare the cell to a normal lymphocyte.

MONOCYTES

Monocytes are the largest normal cell in the peripheral circulation. Their size can make them slightly easier to identify. They are 12 to 30 μm in diameter. Their nucleus is irregular or "brain shaped," with the folds giving the appearance of convolutions. The chromatin is loose, forming a pattern that looks like old-fashioned lace. The cytoplasm is homogeneous with a fine speckled appearance, like "ground glass." The monocyte's primary function is to phagocytize bacteria, fungi, degenerating blood cells, and products of tissue damage. Monocytes also process antigens.

The electron microscope has shown that there are two forms of granules in the cytoplasm. One type is similar to the lysosomes of the neutrophil. The function of the other is not presently known. The granules similar to lysosomes are called **azurophilic** (primary) **granules** and have their origin on the inner membranes of the organelle called the Golgi bodies. When using the electron microscope, the presence of these granules in electron micrographs (microscopic pictures) illustrates the common origin of these various groups of cells.

Monocytes can appear smaller than expected and can assume different shapes. They are not always easy to differentiate from larger lymphocytes. (Refer to Figure 4.1 for the morphology of this cell.)

THE MONOCYTIC CELL LINE

The monocytic cell line has as its most mature cell the monocyte. In the most mature state the monocyte can leave the circulation, entering the body tissues and becoming a wandering macrophage (a large eating cell).

The series begins with a blast form, as in most other cell lines. The blast is known as the *monoblast*. The monoblast is a large cell with a diameter of 15 to 20 μm. This cell has a nuclear/cytoplasmic ratio of 4:1 and has a round nucleus with up to four nucleoli present. The nucleus may be centrally located or may be off center (eccentric) and may even be slightly folded in on itself. The scant cytoplasm there is stains blue, but not dark blue, and is agranular. It can be difficult to distinguish between this cell and the myeloblast. Special stains must be used to distinguish between the monoblast and the myeloblast. Identification of leukemia type depends on this distinction. Monoblasts have little, if any, peroxidase; therefore, they have a negative or very weakly positive reaction to the stain. Myeloblasts have a strong reaction to the stain. These cells are never normally in the peripheral circulation, as with other cell line blast forms. These cells are positive for nonspecific esterase stains.

The second stage is the *promonocyte*. They are just a little larger than the blast form, about 14 to 22 μm in diameter. The nucleus/cytoplasmic ratio is 3:1 and the chromatin is slightly more condensed. The promonocyte may also show a lacy open appearance, which helps identify them in the bone marrow. There

---

E X E R C I S E  **IDENTIFICATION OF MONOCYTES**

SAFETY TECHNIQUE: WEAR GLOVES.

Purpose: Identification of monocytes is essential for accurately reading a differential slide.

Equipment Needed: Blood smears provided by the instructor.

Procedure:
1. Using the oil immersion lens (100×), bring the smear into focus.
2. Locate the thin area of the smear.
3. Locate cells identified as a monocyte and make a drawing of them. Notice their size relative to all other cells in the vicinity of the monocyte.

are usually less nucleoli in the nucleus, and many cells show as central fold. They are not normally seen in the peripheral circulation. The cytoplasm is bluish grey in color and some very small purple granules may be seen. The cytoplasm also has irregular blunt pseudopods (small extensions of the cytoplasm).

THE MEGAKARYOCYTIC SERIES

The development of cell fragments called **platelets** begins with the **megakaryocyte** cells. Although not considered white blood cells, some classifications consider these cells agranulocytic. They will also be discussed in Unit 8, which considers hemostasis.

Megakaryocytes reside in the bone marrow and are under the control of the hormone thrombopoietin. Their cytoplasm breaks off in maturation to produce platelets, also called *thrombocytes*. These thrombocytes are released into the blood vessels and initiate primary and secondary hemostasis, discussed in Unit 8.

The first committed cell in this cell line is called the *megakaryoblast*. It is similar to other blast forms in that it is large (approximately 24 µm in diameter) with a rounded nucleus and visible nucleoli. This cell also has basophilic staining in the cytoplasm, with a large nucleus/cytoplasm ratio.

The *promegakaryocyte* is the next stage of development in which there are clearly visible azurophilic granules that start near the nucleus. The nucleus has visible lobes at this time and the cell is about 14 to 30 µm in diameter. The third stage in the development of megakaryocytes is a cell with an increase in the granulation seen in the cytoplasm, called the stage III megakaryocyte. It is larger still, being 16 to 50 µm in diameter. The fourth stage in the development of megakaryocytes is a stage IV megakaryocyte, having a compacted nucleus. The cytoplasm is totally pink. Some authors do not list stage IV as being different from the granular megakaryocyte of stage III.

The mature megakaryocytes are close to bone marrow sinuses, for easy entrance into the bloodstream by the thrombocytes. They have seven to eight masses of cytoplasm around them that are forming thrombocytes.

The megakaryocytic line can be observed in a hematology reference textbook. The laboratory scientist rarely (if ever) sees a megakaryocyte. Platelet identification is of primary importance to the hematologist.

READING THE DIFFERENTIAL SMEAR

If the differential smear is properly made, it will have an area where the cells are covering one another and an area in which the cells do not touch each other. If the correctly made slide is held up to the light, the edge of the slide can show yellows, reds, or orange colors when viewed against a light source. This feathered area is the area of choice in reading a differential count. Review the *Differential Staining* section in Unit 3 concerning staining the slide for a differential. Exercise 48 is performed to begin to obtain skills needed to successfully complete a differential count.

EXERCISE  IDENTIFICATION OF MEGAKARYOCYTES AND PLATELETS

SAFETY TECHNIQUE: WEAR GLOVES.

Purpose: Identification of megakaryocytes helps in understanding the origin of platelets and the coagulation process.

Equipment Needed: Bone marrow smears provided by the instructor, peripheral blood smears.

Procedure:

1. Using the low power objective (10×), bring a bone marrow smear into focus.
2. Using the mechanical stage apparatus, move around the smear to locate the largest cells on the smear. These very large cells are the megakaryocytes. Check with your instructor to make sure that you are looking at the correct cells.
3. Switch to high power (45×) and move the objective toward the oil immersion lens (100×). Do not engage the lens.
4. Place a drop of immersion oil on the smear and engage the oil immersion lens. Readjust the focus if necessary.
5. Look for the presence of small pieces of cytoplasm pinching off to form thrombocytes. Make a drawing of the megakaryocyte.
6. Under oil immersion, look at a normal peripheral blood smear. Locate the platelets. Ask your instructor to verify that you are seeing the platelets.

In some disease states, the amount of immature cells increases in numbers. This is called a "shift to the left" when an increase in immature granulocytes is seen. This is seen most commonly when band cells (Exercise 40) are increased in the peripheral circulation, often accompanying an infection in the patient.

CELL IDENTIFICATION

When identifying white blood cells, the following inquiries are helpful.

- Look at the cytoplasm. What color is it? Are there recognizable granules? If not, it is probably not a granulocyte.
- Observe the nucleus. Are there different lobes in the nucleus? If so, how many lobes are seen in the nucleus? If the cell has observable lobes, it is probably a granulocyte.
- Compare the size of the cell to the red blood cells. If it is close in size to the red blood cell, it may be a lymphocyte. If it is larger than all other cells in the field, it may be a monocyte.

(Figure 4.9 is a leukocyte identification key that can help in the identification of white blood cells while performing the differential count.)

Cell Monocyte	Eosinophil	Basophil	PMN	Band form	Lymphocyte
Nucleus Brain shaped (1)	Lobed (2)	Lobed (2)	Lobed (3)	Ribbon shaped (1 continuous)	Round (1)
Cytoplasm Large amount No granules Greyish color	Red granules	Dark blue granules	Neutral/ lilac granules	Red/blue/lilac granules	Absent/ present

fig. 4.9. Leukocyte identification key.

EXERCISE 48 THE DIFFERENTIAL COUNT

Purpose: To identify the various types of cells found when observing 100 white blood cells using oil immersion microscopy.

Equipment Needed: Compound light microscope, prepared blood smears, immersion oil, and differential counter.

Procedure:

1. Holding a properly labeled and stained slide, observe for the feathered edge. Place this slide on the microscope stage. Apply the mechanical slide holders.

2. Bring the slide into focus under the low power objective. Scan the slide for distribution of cells.

3. Apply a drop of oil to the feathered edge. It is imperative to view the slide in this area, where cells are neither too sparse nor too crowded.

4. Bring the oil immersion lens into position, making sure that the other objectives do not pass through the oil on the slide.

5. See if the red blood cells just touch each other. If they do not, move the mechanical stage until they do.

6. Observe the slide to note the presence or absence of platelets. Red cell morphology will be discussed in Units 6 and 7.

7. Using the pattern shown in Figure 4.10, start identifying the white blood cells and recording them on the differential counter. Most individuals find that using the first two fingers to signify neutrophils and lymphocytes is the easiest method. The ring finger and little finger are generally used for monocytes, eosinophils, and basophils.

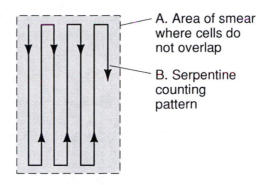

fig. 4.10. Pattern to perform a differential count. (From Marshall. *Fundamental Skills for the Clinical Laboratory Professional.* p. 359.)

It is advisable to commit to memory the normal counts for the major white cells seen in the normal differential (see Table 4.2). This allows for a comparison with other differentials. Often laboratories develop their own normals, given their individual populations. If this is the case, adapt to the levels established by the employer.

ABNORMAL WHITE BLOOD CELLS

Certain disease states cause abnormal cells in the peripheral circulation. Some abnormal cells are discussed below. For a more complete treatment of this important topic, refer to a hematology reference textbook.

LE CELLS

Systemic lupus erythematosus (SLE) is an autoimmune disorder where the patient's immune system attacks the patient. In the past, diagnosis of this disease came from identification of an LE cell, abnormal segmented neutrophil, or other phagocytic cell with the engulfed homogeneous and swollen nucleus of either a neutrophil or lymphocyte. This test has been replaced by the *antinuclear antibody (ANA)* procedure because of its greater sensitivity.

REED-STERNBERG CELLS

Reed-Sternberg cells are found in the lymph nodes. They are often found in association with Hodgkin's disease, a malignant disease of lymphatic cells. They are

Table 4.2. Normal Values for Leukocytes

Adult polys (neutrophils)	50%–70%
Lymphocytes (B & T cells)	20%–35%
Monocytes	2%–6%
Neutrophilic band cells	2%–5%
Eosinophils	0%–3%
Basophils	0%–1%

very large cells, being about five times the size of a neutrophil. They have a multilobed nucleus with several RBC-sized nucleoli that stain light blue in color.

HAIRY CELLS

Hairy cells are a form of B-lymph chronic leukemia, more common in males than in females. The cells are so named because of the projections from the plasma membrane that look like fine hairs.

MOTT CELLS

Mott cells, also called "grape cells," are plasma cells with inclusions called Russell bodies. The inclusions may be transparent sacs staining bluish. It appears as if grape clusters are within the cell.

FLAME CELLS

Flame cells are plasma cells in which the cytoplasm stains a bright red in color, most often associated with IgA myeloma.

SMUDGE CELLS

Smudge cells are the bare nucleus of crushed lymphocytes or other cells. These cells are produced during the smearing process of slide making. A large number of smudge cells may be seen in certain leukemias. Their presence may indicate the increased fragility of the cells. These cells should not be counted in the differential.

SUMMARY

Correct white blood cell identification is an extremely important task for the hematologist. The functions of white blood cells (leukocytes) are diverse and numerous. In contrast to red blood cells (erythrocytes), leukocytes primarily function outside blood vessels. Changes in either function or number of leukocytes reflect a definite change in the body's function, providing important diagnostic information.

Blood cells have their origins in an undifferentiated cell called a stem cell. White blood cells are divided into granulocytic and agranulocytic categories. Granulocytes develop from myeloblasts, maturing from the blast stage to the promyelocyte, the myelocyte, and the metamyelocyte. The band stage is the next stage, with the most mature forms being neutrophils, eosinophils, and basophils. Granulocytes (primarily the neutrophil) provide the first line of defense against invasion from bacteria. Eosinophils and basophils function to suppress inflammation in the body tissues and are implicated in allergic reactions as well as in other functions.

Agranulocytes include lymphocytes, monocytes, and megakaryocytes (precursors to platelets). Lymphocytes are involved with the immune system and its response to invading organisms. There are many types of lymphocytes, including the T-lymphocyte and the B-lymphocyte. Atypical lymphocytes are lymphocytes that are actually stimulated T-lymphocytes seen in viral infections, including infectious mononucleosis, infectious hepatitis, and so on.

Monocytes are the largest normal cell in the peripheral circulation. They function to phagocytize bacteria, fungi, and other degenerating products. They also process antigens. The megakaryocytic series, although not classified as white blood cells, are called agranulocytes. Megakaryocytic cells originate in the bone marrow. Their cytoplasm breaks off in maturation to produce platelets (thrombocytes), which initiate primary and secondary hemostasis.

Differential smear readings are critically important in identifying such abnormalities as infections, leukemias, and other disease states. In order to clearly identify 100 white blood cells and calculate the percentages of each present, a correctly made side is critical. Proper cell identification takes much practice and patience. Abnormal white blood cells that might be seen in a differential include Reed-Sternberg cells, hairy cells, Mott cells, flame cells, and smudge cells.

REVIEW QUESTIONS

1. From among the following, which is characterized by a dark blue cytoplasm, nucleoli, and homogenous chromatin?
   a. myeloblast
   b. lymphoblast
   c. monoblast
   d. all of the above
2. Multilobed cells with little granulation found in large quantities in the differential count are called
   a. T-lymphocytes
   b. neutrophils
   c. monocytes
   d. B-lymphocytes
3. Which cells are considered immature in the peripheral circulation?
   a. erythrocytes
   b. neutrophils
   c. eosinophils
   d. monocytes
4. Which of the following cells is associated with allergic reactions?
   a. neutrophils
   b. monocytes
   c. lymphocytes
   d. basophils
5. Is the presence of band neutrophils normal in the differential? If so, how many would be considered normal?
   a. no, 0
   b. yes, 0 to 1
   c. yes, 0 to 5
   d. yes, 15 to 35

6. You have a slide that has 37% lymphocytes—is this normal?
   a. it is a normal amount
   b. it is below the normal amount
   c. it is slightly elevated above the normal amount
   d. it is greatly elevated above the normal amount

7. The cell you are looking at in the differential count is very large with a greyish cytoplasm and a convoluted nucleus. It is
   a. an atypical lymphocyte
   b. a monocyte
   c. a basophil
   d. an eosinophil

8. The primitive stem cell is also called the
   a. colony-forming unit
   b. hemocytoblast
   c. erythroblast
   d. unidentified colony unit

9. Of the following, which are normally found in the peripheral circulation?
   a. monocytes
   b. megakaryocytes
   c. myeloblasts
   d. metamyelocytes

10. Of the following, which is characterized by an indented nucleus?
    a. myeloblast
    b. promyelocyte
    c. myelocyte
    d. metamyelocyte

11. Of the following, which is the immediate precursor of the PMN?
    a. promyelocyte
    b. metamyelocyte
    c. band cell
    d. myelocyte

12. If pernicious anemia is present, there can be an increase in this type of cell.
    a. neutrophils
    b. bands
    c. metamyelocytes
    d. hypersegmented PMNs

13. The numbers of this cell greatly increase in parasitic infections.
    a. neutrophils
    b. basophils
    c. eosinophils
    d. lymphocytes

14. This cell has an eccentric nucleus, spoked-wheel appearance, and dark blue cytoplasm.
    a. lymphocyte
    b. atypical lymphocyte
    c. plasmacyte
    d. megakaryocyte

15. The cell usually seen in the differential in infectious mononucleosis is the
    a. eosinophil
    b. basophil
    c. lymphocyte
    d. atypical lymphocyte

16. Which of the following is currently being used to detect infectious mononucleosis?
    a. presumptive heterophil
    b. differential heterophil
    c. guinea pig absorption
    d. Monospot

17. Which of the following is not normally seen in the peripheral circulation?
    a. megakaryocyte
    b. monocyte
    c. neutrophil
    d. lymphocyte

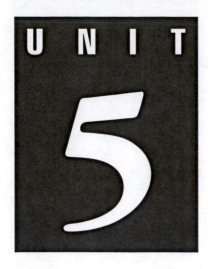

UNIT 5

Leukocyte Abnormalities

LEARNING OBJECTIVES

Having completed this section, it is the responsibility of the student to know the following:

■ Explain a leukemoid reaction.

■ Identify the difference between acute and chronic forms of leukemia.

■ Discuss the various types of leukemia.

■ Describe the cell forms that are used to identify leukemias.

■ Describe the characteristics of multiple myeloma and Hodgkin's disease.

GLOSSARY

acute leukemia condition in which blast forms of a particular cell line are often found in great quantities.

anemia condition in which red blood cells are being destroyed, their ability to carry oxygen is hindered, or red blood cells are being destroyed faster than they are produced.

Auer rods cellular inclusions that stain red with Wright's stain; found in the cytoplasm of myeloblasts of acute myelogenous leukemia.

chronic leukemia condition in which there is an increase in the mature cell line(s).

cytochemical analysis use of staining techniques to identify elements within the cytoplasm of a cell.

-cytosis increase in a cell line.

diurnal daily cycle in the absolute numbers of cells.

hematocrit packed cell volume of a certain amount of blood.

hemoglobin amount of oxygen-carrying capability of the red blood cell.

hepatomegaly increase in the normal size of the liver.

leukopoietins colony-stimulating factors that can increase the reproductivity of various types of white blood cells; also known as growth factors such as G-CSF, GM-CSF, and interleukins.

lymphoma malignant disorder affecting the lymphatic tissues.

monoclonal antibodies specific immune chemicals produced from a single cell origin.

morphology form and structure of organisms.

myelodysplastic syndromes characterized by an abnormal or ineffective blood cell production in two or more cell lines; examples include refractory megaloblastic anemia and chronic myelomonocytic leukemia.

pancytopenia decrease in all blood cell lines.

-penia decrease in a cell line.

prognosis outcome of a disease state.

refractory not readily yielding to treatment.

splenomegaly increase in the size of the spleen.

INTRODUCTION

An increase in the number of white cells is seen in many conditions, including inflammations and infections. These increases can be caused by an overproduction in the bone marrow of a particular cell line. They can also be caused by entrance into circulation of already existing white cells from an area called the marginal pool of the body tissues. The increase is usually designated with the suffix **-cytosis,** as in leuko*cytosis.* A decrease in white cells is designated with the suffix **-penia,** as in neutro*penia.*

MARGINAL AND CIRCULATORY POOLS

The response of the body to its daily challenges and disease states is often an increase in the number of leukocytes. This can be achieved by two means. Increasing the production of cells from the bone marrow can be caused by a secretion of **leukopoietins.** The other way of increasing cells is by placing back into circulation those cells about to leave the bloodstream to enter the body tissues, called the marginal pool.

ABSOLUTE CONCENTRATIONS OF LEUKOCYTES

It sometimes becomes important to know if an increase in a particular white cell is an actual increase. The temporary increase actually might be due to a decrease in other cell lines, artificially increasing a white cell line. Laboratory scientists can calculate the absolute concentration of each type of cell. The total white cell count is multiplied by the percentage of the individual cell line in question.

At birth, some immature white blood cells are present in the peripheral circulation. These immature cells disappear in a few days. The total white blood cell count in a newborn decreases from 10 to $25 \times$ (times) $10^9/L$ to 5 to $15 \times 10^9/L$, remaining at that level up to age 4. It then reaches 4 to $11 \times 10^9/L$ as seen in an adult.

Exercise 49 includes a calculation of the absolute concentrations of white blood cells.

LEUKEMOID REACTIONS

A leukemoid reaction is a bodily response that resembles leukemia but is not leukemia. The distinction between the two states is made by clinical observations of the patient and laboratory testing, including a bone marrow examination and leukocyte alkaline phosphatase stain (LAP). The most common forms are neutrophilic and lymphocytic leukemoid reactions.

The *neutrophilic leukemoid reaction* is a condition accompanied by a high white cell count of up to $100 \times 10^9/L$. The differential usually shows immature cells such as bands, metamyelocytes, and myelocytes. This resembles chronic myelogenous leukemia (CML). The alkaline phosphatase stain (Unit 4) yields an

EXERCISE 49 CALCULATION OF ABSOLUTE WHITE BLOOD CELL CONCENTRATIONS

SAFETY TECHNIQUE: NONE

Purpose: Calculation of absolute white blood cell counts aids in determining if cell count changes are actual or artificial. Refer to Table 5.1 for reference values for white blood cells.

Procedure:
1. Use the following formula for this activity:
   CELL LINE % × TOTAL WBC
2. A white blood cell count has been obtained of 9×10^9/L and a 35% lymphocyte count. Determine the absolute concentration of lymphocytes. Is the lymphocyte count in the normal range?
3. A white blood cell count has been obtained of 3.5×10^9/L and a 35% lymphocyte count. Determine the absolute concentration of lymphocytes. Is this lymphocyte count in the normal range?

Table 5.1. Normal White Blood Cell Counts

Neutrophils	$= 2.0 - 7.0 \times 10^9$/L with **diurnal** variations
Eosinophils	$= 0.35 \times 10^9$/L with dirunal variations
Basophils	$= 0.2 \times 10^9$/L
Lymphocytes	$= 1.5 - 4.0 \times 10^9$/L with lymphocytosis in childhood decreasing to adult
Monocytes	$= 0.2 - 0.8 \times 10^9$/L with monocytosis in first 2 weeks of life

above-normal value in this condition and a below-normal value in CML. Many diseases are associated with a neutrophilic leukemoid reaction, including tuberculosis, pneumonia, malaria, syphilis, severe burns, Hodgkin's disease, and mercury poisoning.

Other nonmalignant changes that can be seen in neutrophils include the following:

Toxic Granulation: Larger than normal granules can be found in the cytoplasm of neutrophils, staining deeply basophilic or blue-black. Their presence is often associated with acute bacterial infections, burns, and drug poisonings.

Döhle bodies: Döhle bodies are round or oval, small, clear light blue staining areas found in the neutrophil cytoplasm. They are remnants of RNA from an earlier stage of neutrophil development. They are often seen in infections, burns, toxic agent reactions, and pregnancy.

Vacuolization: Cytoplasmic vacuolization can develop in leukocytes from the blood being treated with EDTA. Vacuoles are also signs of toxic change and may indicate phagocytosis.

Pelger-Huët Anomaly: This is a benign anomaly seen as a failure of a neutrophil nucleus to segment or form lobes normally. The neutrophil has a band-shaped nucleus or at most two lobes. These cells function normally. This condition must be distinguished from a "shift to the left" of immature band forms as a result of an infection.

May-Hegglin Anomaly: These are large blue inclusion bodies in neutrophils, larger than Döhle bodies. This is an inherited disorder.

Chédiak-Higashi Anomaly: Neutrophils have large amorphous granules in the cytoplasm. Granules may also be seen in lymphocytic and monocytic cytoplasm. The disease is inherited and rare. The cells do not function properly; marrow transplantation may be the treatment of choice for this disease.

Alder-Reilly Anomaly: Heavy and dark azurophilic granulation is observed in neutrophils, eosinophils, and basophils. Rarely the granulation is observed in lymphocytes and monocytes. This is an inherited anomaly.

A *lymphocytic leukemoid reaction* is also accompanied by a high white cell count, as much as 150×10^9/L, with a differential count of 35% to 95% lymphocytes. The distinction again requires clinical observations, laboratory examinations, and a bone marrow examination. Many diseases are associated with this response, including infectious mononucleosis, pertussis, mumps, measles, infectious lymphocytosis, and chickenpox. Infectious mononucleosis can be distinguished by a Monospot® test.

E X E R C I S E  **NEUTROPHILIC ANOMALIES**

Purpose: Neutrophils can have significant morphologic alterations that may or may not be significant.

Procedure:
1. Your instructor will provide you with prestained slides that contain neutrophils with various alterations.
2. Identify as many alterations in the neutrophils that you see on each slide. Be sure to check with your instructor to make sure that you are correctly identifying the alterations.
3. Make drawings of abnormalities that you see.
4. Which abnormalities are significant? Which are not? Are any abnormalities you see an inherited trait?
5. You might want to do further research into other morphologic alternations seen in leukocytes, such as Barr bodies and Auer rods (mentioned later in this unit).

MYELODYSPLASTIC SYNDROMES

Myelodysplastic syndromes (MDS) are characterized by an abnormal or ineffective blood cell production in two or more cell lines, including granulocytic, red blood cell, and megakaryocytic cell lines. The bone marrow of patients suffering from these syndromes may have hypercellularity in the bone marrow and reduced blood cells circulating in the peripheral blood.

MDS usually affects patients over 50 years of age. Many of the syndromes in this category are considered preleukemic, as most patients will eventually progress toward a form of acute leukemia. Younger patients, often those who have received prolonged therapy with cytotoxic drugs or radiation, can also be affected.

Refractory anemia is also considered a myelodysplastic syndrome, characterized by peripheral anemia that resists treatment with conventional approaches. Red blood cells are not produced properly, with reduced immature forms in the bone marrow. There are several forms of refractory anemia, including refractory anemia with ringed sideroblasts and refractory anemia with excess blasts. Chronic myelomonocytic leukemia is also considered a myelodysplastic syndrome.

LEUKEMIA

The leukemias are malignant disorders of the blood-forming tissues—mainly the bone marrow, lymph nodes, and spleen. In leukemia, the blood-forming tissues flood the bloodstream and lymph system with abnormal and immature (sometimes mature cells as well) white blood cells. These cells cannot carry on the normal cells' function of fighting infections. Moreover, they reduce production of red blood cells and platelets. If the disease is untreated, the abnormal cells become dominant and are carried through the body, proliferating outside of the bone marrow in areas such as the spleen and liver. Infections occur, severe anemia results because of lack of red blood cell production, and bruising and hemorrhaging take place due to the lack of platelets.

Leukemias are found in two forms. **Acute leukemia** is characterized by an appearance in the peripheral circulation of the blast as the predominant form (most immature) of the particular cell line involved. Any white blood cell can start to proliferate in this manner, although neutrophils and lymphocytes are the most common cells involved in leukemia.

The other form of leukemia is **chronic leukemia**, characterized by greatly increased numbers of the more mature cell of the cell line involved along with the presence of blasts and other immature cells. Both forms of leukemia have a common characteristic, the unregulated reproduction of cells.

Most leukemias are of a single type, that is, formed by only one cell line. Studies using **monoclonal antibodies** have shown that cells of mixed characteristics are also involved.

In children diagnosed with acute lymphocytic leukemia (the most common leukemia of childhood), the **prognosis** is excellent, and a cure has been realized in many cases. Chronic forms of leukemia can be controlled for many years. Bone marrow transplants have increased the life expectancy of both acute and chronic leukemia patients.

A **lymphoma** is a general term for a group of malignant disorders that affect the lymphatic tissues. The cells that make up the lymphatic tissues become abnormal, multiplying continuously and crowding the normal cells that cannot function properly. Without treatment, lymphomas lead to development of tumors with ultimate invasion of vital organs.

Lymphomas usually are associated with B- or T-lymphocytes and may invade a single node or many locations within the body.

LEUKEMIA IDENTIFICATION TECHNIQUES

There often are two characteristics of leukemias. The white blood cell count is often ten or more times the normal count, and the differential is "shifted to the left," with an increase in immature forms. However, some leukemias will not initially present with a high white blood cell count, but abnormal forms will be seen in the differential. Treatment is dependent upon identification of the abnormal cell line.

Familiarity with blast forms will lessen the difficulty in identifying a particular type of leukemia. This identification process is not the responsibility of one laboratory scientist. Clinical pathologists, physicians (hematologists), and supervisorial staff in the hematology department are often involved in helping laboratory scientists accurately identify leukemic cells. Sometimes blood is sent to reference laboratories outside the health care facility for verification of the identification made. The identification is critical; the treatment differs significantly depending on the type of leukemia found.

Many times it is very difficult to distinguish between various types of blasts. Other means of identification are employed. The observation of the other cells on the slide is sometimes very helpful, noticing "the company the unidentified cell keeps." The use of **cytochemical analysis** is also helpful. Cells are stained to determine specific enzymes or other proteins produced by cellular organelles. This must be done without damaging the cellular **morphology**. Cells produce proteins that are very specific and will only be found in a specific cell or in cells that have been incubated with special substrates.

Those cytochemical techniques that are associated with enzymes include acid and alkaline phosphatase, myeloperoxidase, and esterases. Those cytochemical techniques associated with nonenzymatic stains include Sudan black B (lipid stain), toluidine blue (mucopolysaccharide stain), and periodic acid-Schiff (glycogen stain). Cytochemistry is sometimes aided by the electron microscope. Access to this highly sophisticated equipment is limited. Immunochemical techniques using monoclonal antibodies and cytogenetic assays are also useful. Further details about these techniques can be found in hematology reference textbooks.

THE FRENCH-AMERICAN-BRITISH CLASSIFICATION SYSTEM (FAB)

In 1976, a group of hematologists from France, the United States, and Britain developed a system of classifying acute leukemias. This system is based on the morphological characteristics of the cells on a differential or bone marrow slide. They described two major divisions of acute leukemias: the lymphoblastic and the nonlymphoblastic leukemias. Table 5.2 summarizes the FAB classification.

As medical science progresses, researchers discover more and more information about leukemia. Populations of cells once thought to be uniform are now

Table 5.2. The FAB Classification

Classification	Characteristics
MO myelogenous	Myelogenous blasts without peroxidase staining
M1 myelogenous	Blasts and promyelocytes predominate
M2 myelogenous	Myelogenous cells mature beyond blast and promyelocyte forms
M3 promyelocytic	Promyelocytes predominate in bone marrow
M4 myelomonocytic	Both myelogenous and monocytic cells present, being at least 20% of WBCs
M5 monocytic	Most cells are monocytic; there are two subtypes A. Large blasts in bone marrow and peripheral blood B. Monoblasts, promonocytes, and monocytes
M6 erythroleukemia	Di Guglielmo syndrome: abnormal red cell proliferation and granulocytic precursors
M7 megakaryocytic	Large and small megakaryoblasts
L1 homogeneous	Only one population of cells, small cells predominate, nucleus shape regular, chromatic homogeneous, nucleoli missing, cytoplasm moderately basophilic
L2 heterogeneous	Large cells, nucleus irregular shape, indentations seen in nucleus, one or more nucleoli seen, cytoplasm color varies
L3 Burkitt's lymphoma	Cells large and homogeneous in size, lymphoma nucleus is round to oval, one to three nucleoli easily seen, cytoplasm deeply basophilic, vacuoles often prominent

discovered to be mixed populations. This manual will not discuss in detail all various forms of leukemia. The student is encouraged to read the latest materials about new discoveries and consult hematology reference texts for more in-depth discussions of rarely seen leukemias. This manual will discuss four of the most common forms of leukemia: acute myelogenous leukemia, acute lymphocytic leukemia, chronic myelogenous leukemia, and chronic lymphocytic leukemia. Some other forms will be briefly discussed.

ACUTE MYELOGENOUS LEUKEMIA

Acute myelogenous leukemia (AML) is sometimes also called acute myelocytic leukemia, acute myeloblastic leukemia, acute granulocytic leukemia (AGL), or acute nonlymphocytic leukemia. Acute myelogenous leukemia can be divided into several subtypes, including:

- Acute promyelocytic leukemia (APL)
- Acute myelomonocytic leukemia (AMML)
- Acute monocytic leukemia (AMOL)
- Acute erythroleukemia
- Acute megakaryocytic leukemia

There are slight differences in the prognosis and treatment responses for the various subtypes. This discussion will focus on aspects of AML related to most subtypes. Students are encouraged to read on their own about rare subtypes of AML.

AML is characterized by a great increase in the white blood cell count (see Figure 5.1) and by the presence of myeloblasts in the differential count. The white blood cell count, when normal, is 5 to 10×10^9/L. In AML, 70% of patients have a leukocytosis. The high white cell count may drop to normal or even below normal during a remission of the disease. The normal differential shows an absence of myeloblasts, but myeloblasts can dominate the differential count in AML. The differential also shows a few promyelocytes, myelocytes, and metamyelocytes. Since these early cell forms are usually hard to identify, look for neutrophils, which may be as high as 10% of the differential count. If neutrophils are seen, the cells in question may also be from the same cell line.

The differential count may also show some **Auer rods** in the cytoplasm of the blast forms. These are reddish rods that also can appear in promyelocytes and monoblasts of patients with acute myelogenous leukemia. Peroxidase stain testing is helpful in distinguishing between acute myelogenous (AML) and acute lymphocytic leukemia (ALL), because in acute lymphocytic leukemia 95% to 100% of the cells are peroxidase negative.

Approximately 6400 new cases of AML are diagnosed each year in the United States. AML is usually diagnosed in people over the age of 50. However, it can occur in any age group.

Patients with AML usually complain about being tired and weak, with pains in bones or joints. They can look pale and often note that they bruise easily and develop purplish-red blotches on their skin (called petechiae). Gums and noses may bleed. The spleen often is enlarged (**splenomegaly**), as well as the liver (**hepatomegaly**). Diagnosis can be made by the physician performing a physical examination, blood tests, and a bone marrow sample.

In this and many other types of leukemias, the malignant cell growth can be so great that it crowds out normal cell growth, resulting in a decrease in the red blood cells and platelets. Therefore, **hemoglobin** and **hematocrit** values fall, as do platelet counts, resulting in an **anemic** condition. The differential cell count may contain immature red blood cells due to the body's attempt to produce new cells.

The decreased platelet count can cause bleeding problems. Because of the increased amount of white cells, the blood must be diluted for counting, whether the count is manual or automated.

Treatment for AML is very complex and has risks. A plan for treatment is developed for each patient by hematologists, oncologists, and radiologists trained in the diagnosis and treatment of malignant blood diseases. The goal of the treatment is to induce remission of the disease, where signs and symptoms of the disease cannot be detected. The bone marrow must be found free of any leukemia cells.

Patients younger than 45 can be candidates for a bone marrow transplant, which has been found to have impressive results. *Chemotherapy* is another

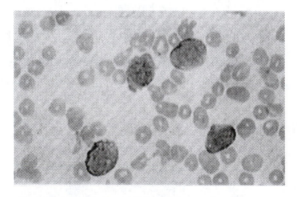

fig. 5.1. Acute myelogenous leukemia. (From Marshall. *Fundamental Skills for the Clinical Laboratory Professional.* p. 330.)

means used to treat AML. Chemotherapy is the use of drugs that kill cancers. Sometimes *radiation* is also used to supplement the chemotherapy.

Exercise 51 is designed to acquaint the student with the immature cells of acute myelogenous leukemia.

ACUTE LYMPHOCYTIC LEUKEMIA

Acute lymphocytic leukemia (ALL) is also known as acute lymphatic, acute lymphoblastic, or acute lymphogenous leukemia. This leukemia is considered the most curable of all major forms of leukemia in children. It is the leading form of leukemia in children, representing approximately 85% of leukemia in patients under 21 (refer to Figure 4.6 in Unit 4).

ALL is primarily diagnosed in children between 2 and 10 years old. It is, however, found in all age groups. There are more than 4000 new cases of ALL reported in the United States each year.

The FAB group has suggested three types of acute lymphocytic leukemia. As research advances are made, these categories are often expanded.

E X E R C I S E **IDENTIFICATION OF ACUTE MYELOGENOUS LEUKEMIA**

Purpose: AML can appear on the differential as having a large number of very early cells, mostly blast forms. Refer to color plates of leukemic cells in a hematology reference textbook.

Procedure:
1. Using the oil immersion lens (100X), bring the smear into focus.
2. Identify a cell that you believe is a myeloblast. Ask your instructor to verify what you are seeing.
3. Make a drawing of the field of vision.
4. See if you can identify other cells, such as promyelocytes, myelocytes, metamyelocytes, bands, and neutrophils. Keep in mind that identification of leukemic cells takes much experience.

Table 5.3. Classification of ALL

Cytological Feature	L1	L2	L3
Amount cytoplasm	Small amount	Variable, often abundant	Moderately abundant
Basophilia	Little/moderate	Variable, deep in some cases	Very deep
Cell size	Small	Large, heterogenous	Large, homogenous
Chromatin	Same in any case	Variable in any case	Finely stippled and homogenous
Nucleoli	Absent	One or more large	Prominent, one or more
Nucleus shape	Regular	Irregular, indented	Regular-oval/round
Vacuolization	Variable	Variable	Prominent

Symptoms of ALL include frequent infections and influenza-like symptoms such as high fever, chills, and respiratory discomfort. Weakness and irritability due to anemia are common. Swollen lymph nodes occur frequently, particularly in children. The liver or spleen can become enlarged, causing the abdomen to protrude. As with AML, bleed problems may occur in ALL, causing small cuts to bleed profusely, menstrual periods to be unusually heavy, and blood to appear in the stool. Petechiae can also be present on the skin, with gum and nosebleeds a problem as well.

Diagnosis involves laboratory testing, with a leukocytosis often appearing, the total leukocyte count being most commonly between 5×10^9/L and 25×10^9/L. The differential illustrates lymphoblasts and usually "smudge cells," which are not counted. The presence of these abnormal cellular conditions indicates the fragility of the cells involved. The peroxidase stain shows a negative result. The differential also shows decreased platelets, red cells, and some nucleated (immature) red blood cells.

Treatment of ALL can include bone marrow transplantation and chemotherapy. Central nervous system prophylaxis is used to target brain and spinal column involvement in this leukemia. There has been a dramatic improvement in survival rates for all ages suffering from ALL.

Use of Monoclonal Antibodies in Classification

The use of monoclonal antibodies has helped the classification process of ALL. The most common form of ALL has acute lymphocytic leukemia antigen (CALLA) associated with surface markers on the red blood cells. The T-ALL subgroup has been identified by the presence of T-cell markers. The B-ALL subgroup has been identified by membrane surface markers or by the presence of cytoplasmic/surface membrane immunoglobulin. This is the rarest form of ALL.

A null cell or unclassified ALL has been identified because of the lack of surface markers. This leukemia is associated with a poor prognosis.

As well as using monoclonal antibodies, it has also been found that some intracellular enzymes may also have importance in classifying ALL. The enzyme TdT is detected by direct enzyme testing or indirectly by using immunofluorescence. This enzyme is not normally found in lymphocytes but can be found in the cortex of the thymic population of lymphocytes (about 65% of the cells found there). In ALL, the presence of this enzyme confirms CALLA and T-ALL.

Chromosome Abnormalities in ALL

About 15% of children affected by ALL have the presence of the Philadelphia chromosome (Ph[1]), which has been associated with a poor prognosis. This chromosome has also been found in adults with ALL. This is a translocation of one arm of a chromosome to another chromosome. About 50% of the ALL cases have some abnormalities in the chromosomes. Chromosome analysis is an important tool in predicting treatment outcome in ALL.

RARE FORMS OF ACUTE LEUKEMIAS

The following types of leukemia are very rare and are listed here for reference.

- **Acute eosinophilic leukemia** is considered by many researchers to be a variant of chronic myelogenous leukemia. It can resemble reactive eosinophilia or CML.

E X E R C I S E 52 **IDENTIFICATION OF ACUTE LYMPHOCYTIC LEUKEMIA**

Purpose: Acute lymphocytic leukemia is characterized by the presence of immature lymphocytes, mainly lymphoblasts.

Equipment Needed: Blood smears provided by the instructor.

Procedure:
1. Using the oil immersion lens (100X), bring the smear into focus.
2. Locate a lymphoblast. Ask your instructor to verify what you see.
3. Make a drawing of the field of vision.
4. Observe other cells in the field.
5. Consult a hematology reference textbook for more examples of ALL.

- **Stem cell leukemia** is diagnosed when the blast cells seen in the differential count are so immature that they cannot be identified as to the exact cell line. As the disease progresses, the cells become mature enough to become identified as to cell line, and a final diagnosis can be made at that time. This rare disorder is usually found in children.
- **Basophilic leukemia** is possibly the rarest form of leukemia, usually occurring in middle-aged males. The most significant characteristic is the presence of 50% to 80% basophils in the differential smear.

CHRONIC LEUKEMIAS

Chronic forms of leukemia are characterized by an increase in the numbers of more mature cells of a particular cell line. There is also an increase in the total leukocyte count. There are two common forms of chronic leukemias: chronic myelogenous leukemia and chronic lymphocytic leukemia.

Chronic Myelogenous Leukemia

Chronic myelogenous leukemia (CML) is also called chronic granulocytic leukemia, chronic myelocytic leukemia, chronic myelosis, or chronic myeloid leukemia. It accounts for approximately 25% of all leukemias. It is primarily considered an "adult" leukemia because it usually occurs in individuals between 30 and 50 years old. CML is found in people of all ages, but it is very unusual for children and adolescents to develop this disease.

Five subtypes have been identified:

1. The common type
2. Juvenile CML—occurs from 0 to 5 years of age
3. Chronic neutrophilic leukemia
4. Chronic myelomonocytic leukemia
5. Atypical CML—considered to be intermediate between subtypes 1 and 4

Like other leukemias, symptoms of this disease include complaints attributed to anemia, with feelings of weakness, fatigue, dizziness, headaches, and irritability. The spleen often becomes enlarged, and excessive bleeding is common. In its early stages, the patient is often without symptoms. This disease is often discovered accidentally during a routine physical examination.

The total leukocyte count can be 100 to 800×10^9/L, achieving the highest levels of all leukemias. This count may drop to normal or even below normal with treatment or remission or in the terminal phase. The differential count shows a predominance of myelocytes (20% to 50%), but all cells of the series can be seen. The amount of basophils may also increase up to 12%. There will be a decrease in red blood cell production, and nucleated red cells can be found in the differential, with oddly shaped (poikilocytosis) red blood cells present. There is a decrease in the alkaline phosphatase stain value. Platelets may be increased at the start of the disease, but usually fall to normal or decrease in the terminal stages. The abnormal Philadelphia chromosome is found in this disease.

Bone marrow transplantation has been very successful in this leukemia. Interferon is a glycoprotein that is used frequently in the treatment of this disease. Chemotherapy is also used.

Patients can live for years, relatively symptom-free, in the initial stages of this leukemia. It can be easily controlled with mild chemotherapeutic drugs. The leukemia can, however, recur and become more resistant. The leukemia can convert into an acute phase where blasts are pushed into the bloodstream.

Chronic Lymphocytic Leukemia

Chronic lymphocytic leukemia (CLL) is also known as chronic lymphatic, chronic lymphogenous, or chronic lymphoid leukemia. It is the most common of all

---

E X E R C I S E **IDENTIFICATION OF CHRONIC MYELOGENOUS LEUKEMIA**

Purpose: Chronic myelogenous leukemia is characterized by increases in all lines of cells, with immature red and white blood cells often present as well.

Equipment Needed: Blood smears provided by the instructor.

Procedure:
1. Using the oil immersion lens (100X), bring the smear into focus, focusing first on low power.
2. Observe the wide variety of cells you see in the field of vision.
3. Attempt to do a 100-cell differential count on this slide. It is often possible to complete the differential by observing very few fields.
4. Ask your instructor to help you identify immature cells. A hematology reference textbook with color plates is very helpful when observing leukemia slides.
5. Draw a field of vision.

leukemias in Western countries, accounting for approximately 30% of all reported cases. It is extremely rare among Eastern nations.

At least 8600 new cases are diagnosed annually in the United States. This is a disease of middle or old age, although this leukemia has occurred at other ages. At diagnosis approximately 90% of all CLL patients are over 50, with the incidence increasing with age. Two-thirds of the affected patients are men.

The total leukocyte count is 50 to 200×10^9/L and may drop in remission, chemotherapy, or the terminal stages of the disease. The differential count shows an increase in the number of lymphocytes from a normal of 20% to 35% to 75% to 95%. Initially the platelet count and RBC production may be normal, but later they are decreased. Nucleated red blood cells are commonly seen in the differential.

The pace of untreated CLL varies considerably from patient to patient. Some patients may take 20 years to have the disease progress to a life-threatening point. Chemotherapy is successful against this leukemia and is often not used until the patient is symptomatic.

OTHER CHRONIC LEUKEMIAS

- **Chronic myelomonocytic leukemia** is a disease of old age; patients are often diagnosed while being examined for other conditions. Patients may present with bruising or symptoms of anemia, and there may be an enlarged spleen. The white blood cell count is usually increased, but in some cases it is normal or decreased. A monocytosis is characteristically present with abnormal "U-shaped" nuclei.
- **Plasmacytic leukemia** is a very rare disease. Some researchers suggest that it is only a terminal stage in multiple myeloma. The total leukocyte count is

EXERCISE   **IDENTIFICATION OF CHRONIC LYMPHOCYTIC LEUKEMIA**

SAFETY TECHNIQUE: WEAR GLOVES.

Purpose: Chronic lymphocytic leukemia is characterized by the presence of numerous mature lymphocytes.

Equipment Needed: Blood smears provided by the instructor.

Procedure:
1. Using the oil immersion lens (100X) bring the smear into focus, starting with low power.
2. Observe for the presence of the malignant mature lymphocytes that characterize CLL.
3. Draw a field of vision.

between 20 and 60 × 10⁹/L, and the differential count shows a rise in plasma cells from a normal of 0% to 25% to 90%.

- **Hairy cell leukemia** (Figure 5.2) is a disorder seen predominantly in males (male to female ratio: 7:1). The typical patient has a prominent splenomegaly. The differential count shows a **pancytopenia** (a decrease in all cell lines). The "hairy" cells appear as large lymphs with cytoplasmic projections. They have a single round or folded nucleus with homogenous chromatin and a single nucleolus. The cytoplasm is light-blue and is usually vacuolated. Treatment with agents such as interferon have shown significantly positive results.

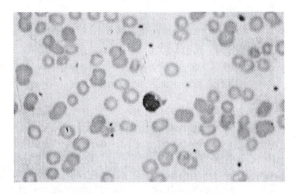

fig. 5.2. Hairy cell leukemia. (From Marshall. *Fundamental Skills for the Clinical Laboratory Professional.* p. 332.)

- **Multiple myeloma** (Figure 5.3) is a condition characterized by many tumors in the bone marrow. The tumors involve the plasma cells to produce excessive abnormal amounts of proteins that can be seen in protein electrophoresis testing (usually carried out in the clinical chemistry department). This disease is usually found in males past age 50. There are small masses in the bones of the shoulders, ribs, and backbone. The destruction of bone causes blood calcium levels to increase. Excessive proteins cause red blood cells to clump together in a rouleau formation (like stacked coins). New treatments, primarily chemotherapy, are adding years to survival rates.

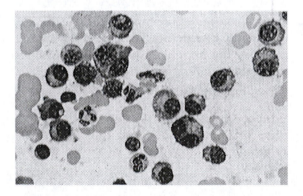

fig. 5.3. Multiple myeloma. (From Marshall. *Fundamental Skills for the Clinical Laboratory Professional.* p. 335.)

55 **IDENTIFICATION OF ROULEAU FORMATION AND PLASMA CELLS IN MULTIPLE MYELOMA**

Purpose: Rouleau formation is formed by increased proteins, and the presence of plasma cells is an indication of multiple myeloma.

Equipment Needed: Blood smears provided by the instructor.

Procedure:
1. Using the oil immersion lens (100X), bring the smear into focus.
2. Observe for the presence of a rouleau formation and plasma cells. Please consult with your instructor if you have questions about identifying these two phenomena.
3. Make a drawing of the field of vision.

Note: Rouleau formation may cause problems when counting red blood cells. The blood may have to be diluted and warmed before testing.

- **Hodgkin's disease** is a malignancy of the lymph system, a common form of lymphoma. This disease usually starts with an enlargement of the lymphatic tissue of the neck and then spreads throughout the body. The disease is characterized by the presence of a type of cell found in the lymph nodes called a Reed-Sternberg cell. This cell is much larger than the typical PMN and is multinuclear. Hodgkin's disease affects all ages and sexes, with the peak concentration of patients being in their 20's to mid-30's. Usually the patient is tired and has chills and sweats. There is an intense itching sensation. Treatment is usually by chemotherapy or X-rays to destroy the tumors. This malignancy can now be arrested in almost 90% of the cases diagnosed in early stages. Students can refer to hematology reference textbooks to research other types of lymphomas.

EXERCISE **56** **IDENTIFICATION OF HODGKIN'S DISEASE**

Purpose: The Reed-Sternberg cell is identified in lymph node biopsies and can appear in the bone marrow of about 10% of patients with Hodgkin's disease.

Equipment Needed: Histology slides provided by the instructor.

Procedure:
1. Using the oil immersion lens (100X), bring the smear into focus, focusing on low power first, as always.
2. Find an example of a Reed-Sternberg cell. Have your instructor verify your findings.
3. Make a drawing of the field of vision.

SUMMARY

An increase in the number of white blood cells in the blood circulation is seen in many disease states, including inflammation and infection. The increase is termed leukocytosis. A decrease is called leukopenia. The response of the body to daily challenges and disease states is often an increase in leukocyte production. Some increases are temporary, and others may indicate a disease process.

A leukemoid reaction is a bodily response that resembles leukemia but is not leukemia. A neutrophilic leukemoid reaction can be caused by diseases such as tuberculosis, pneumonia, malaria, and other maladies. Neutrophils can also have changes within their cells that can be indicative of a disorder, acquired or hereditary. Such anomalies include toxic granulation, Döhle bodies, and vacuolization. A lymphocytic leukemoid reaction can be caused by such viral diseases as infectious mononucleosis, pertussis, mumps, and measles.

Myelodysplastic syndromes are characterized by an abnormal or ineffective blood cell production in two or more cell lines. Many patients with these syndromes, which include refractory anemia and chronic myelomonocytic leukemia, can eventually develop an acute form of leukemia.

Leukemias are a group of diseases involving the malignant proliferation of blood cells. Acute forms (both myelogenous and lymphocytic) are characterized by the appearance of immature blast forms in the peripheral circulation. Chronic leukemias (both myelogenous and lymphocytic) generally have malignancies of mature cell lines as well as immature cells. Identification techniques require cooperation among laboratory scientists, pathologists, hematologists, and supervisorial staff in the hematology department. Cytochemical techniques and immunochemical techniques are often used to categorize leukemias.

Types of leukemia discussed in this unit include acute myelogenous leukemia, acute lymphocytic leukemia, chronic myelogenous leukemia, and chronic lymphocytic leukemia. All of these leukemias, in addition to other less frequently occurring leukemias, have specific characteristics that give the laboratory scientist valuable clues to identification of the leukemia. Exact identification is critical for the proper treatment regimen to effect a remission in the patient.

Other abnormal leukocyte disease states include multiple myeloma and Hodgkin's disease. Multiple myeloma is a condition characterized by many tumors in the bone marrow. The tumors involve the plasma cells that produce excessive and abnormal amounts of proteins. Hodgkin's disease is a malignancy of the lymph system, a common form of lymphoma.

REVIEW QUESTIONS

1. The Philadelphia chromosome (Ph¹) is associated with:
   a. chromic myelogenous leukemia
   b. chronic lymphocytic leukemia
   c. Di Guglielmo's syndrome
   d. multiple myeloma

2. A peripheral smear showing an increase in small lymphocytes with "smudge cells" would indicate the possibility of
   a. multiple myeloma
   b. chronic lymphocytic leukemia
   c. chronic myelogenous leukemia
   d. infectious mononucleosis

3. In Hodgkin's disease, one may find
   a. lymphocytopenia
   b. eosinophilia and neutrophilia
   c. monocytosis
   d. all of the above

4. In chronic myelogenous leukemia, there is
   a. leukopenia
   b. lymphocytosis
   c. marked leukocytosis
   d. basopenia

5. In chronic lymphocytic leukemia, there is
   a. a thrombocythemia
   b. a proliferation of blast forms
   c. increased myelocytes
   d. marked lymphocytosis

6. In acute leukemias, there is generally
   a. thrombocythemia
   b. a normal platelet count
   c. normal clot retraction
   d. a low platelet count

7. Auer rods are seen in the cytoplasm of
   a. myeloblasts
   b. lymphoblasts
   c. megaloblasts
   d. plasma cells

8. Which one of the following cells is considered diagnostic of Hodgkin's disease?
   a. Gaucher's cell
   b. Niemann-Pick cell
   c. atypical lymphocyte
   d. Reed-Sternberg cell

9. Terminal deoxyribonucleotidyl transferase (TdT) is usually found in cells in which of the following?
   a. acute lymphocytic leukemia (ALL)
   b. chronic lymphocytic leukemia (CLL)
   c. chronic myelogenous leukemia (CML)
   d. acute myelogenous leukemia (AML)

10. The most common type of chronic lymphocytic leukemia in the United States is
    a. B cell
    b. null cell
    c. T cell
    d. plasma cell

11. Acute myelogenous leukemia
    a. has no treatment
    b. is never preceded by a preleukemia stage
    c. is often related to immunoglobulin abnormalities
    d. can be differentiated from ALL when myeloblasts contain Auer rods

12. In CML, which of the following is often seen?
    a. increased basophil count
    b. decrease in alkaline phosphatase activity
    c. Philadelphia chromosome
    d. all of the above

13. The type of leukemia most commonly seen in children is
    a. acute monocytic
    b. acute myeloblastic
    c. acute myelomonocytic
    d. acute lymphoblastic

14. This leukemia has a 7:1 male/female ratio, shows a pancytopenia, and the cells have projections.
    a. Hodgkin's disease
    b. Di Guglielmo's syndrome
    c. chronic lymphocytic leukemia
    d. hairy cell leukemia

15. Blast cells appear so immature that they cannot be identified. This leukemia is classified as
    a. stem cell leukemia
    b. hairy cell leukemia
    c. basophilic leukemia
    d. none of the above

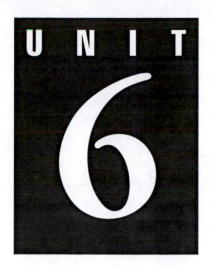

UNIT 6

Red Blood Cells (Erythrocytes)

LEARNING OBJECTIVES

Having completed this unit, it is the responsibility of the student to know the following:

- Describe erythrocytic maturation and destruction.

- Discuss the erythrocyte membrane's structure, function, and abnormalities.

- Describe some abnormal erythrocytic inclusions.

- Discuss the structure of hemoglobin.

- Identify normal hemoglobin and hematocrit levels.

- Describe how a sedimentation rate is performed.

- Calculate red blood cell indices.

GLOSSARY

acidophilic accepting the acid stain eosin, which is red.

anisocytosis variation in the size of the red cells.

basophilic accepting a basic stain, methylene blue, which is blue.

erythropoiesis process by which the hormone erythropoietin is excreted by the kidneys, causing an increased production of RBCs.

femtoliter unit of measure of volume expressed as a portion of a liter; one quadrillionth (10^{-15}) of a liter.

hypochromia having less than the normal color, as seen in anemia.

macrocytes larger than normal cells.

merozoite asexual form of multiplication in malarial parasites.

microcytes smaller than normal cells.

mitotic pool group of early cells capable of cellular mitosis, usually the first two or three cells within the cell line.

picograms unit of measure of weight expressed in grams; one trillionth (10^{-12}) grams.

Plasmodium single-celled flagellate that is the causative agent of malaria.

poikilocytosis alteration in the shape of red cells.

polychromatophilia seen in red cell morphology examination, when red cells stain bluish because of remaining RNA from the immature cell.

pyknotic degeneration of a cell in which the nucleus shrinks in size and the chromatin condenses.

RDW red blood cell distribution width; coefficient of variation of the red blood cell volume distribution, a calculated value on automated cell counters.

sedimentation rate test to determine rate of fall of red blood cells in a glass tube over 1 hour.

sporozoites infecting agent of the malarial parasite.

trophozoite active stage of a malarial parasite.

vector means of transporting of infectious agents.

INTRODUCTION

The erythrocyte was one of the first microscopic structures recognized and described after the development of the microscope. It was not until 1865, however, that the ability to carry oxygen in the red pigment (the heme portion of the hemoglobin molecule) was understood. The red blood cell is about 7 μ in diameter, approximately the same size as a lymphocyte nucleus. A number of disease states are recognized as being exclusively erythrocytic in nature.

ERYTHROCYTE MATURATION

The process by which erythrocytes are created is called **erythropoiesis**. Erythropoiesis is normally an orderly process through which the peripheral concentration of red cells is maintained in a steady state.

Erythrocytic development begins with the cells in the yolk sac of the developing embryo, called the blood islets. These cells increase their mitotic divisions until primitive blood vessels have been formed. Then cells within the center of the primitive vessels either break apart to create the first plasma or become the primitive red blood cells. Cell production continues to take place outside the bone marrow in the liver but ultimately is localized in the spongy bone (cancellous) of the bone marrow in the last trimester of prenatal life and continues in this position throughout adult life.

At birth and thereafter, when a decreased oxygen level enters the kidneys through normal circulation, the hormone erythropoietin is released into the bloodstream. This hormone stimulates the committed erythroid stem cell (CFU-E) units. This results in the increased production of red cells.

Differentiation and maturation takes place in the bone marrow. Maturation takes place over the next 5 to 7 days in the bone marrow. With the expulsion of the nucleus from the red cells, the cells are ready to enter the peripheral circulation. At this stage, they are called erythrocytes, more accurately called reticulocytes. The clinical laboratory scientists could, therefore, determine the rate of production of red cells by observing the number of reticulocytes in the peripheral circulation and counting them (the reticulocyte count). Reticulocytes become mature red cells after about 1 day in peripheral circulation.

Mature red cells have a limited life span of about 120 days (±20 days) and then are removed from circulation by the liver and spleen.

THE RUBRIBLAST

The earliest recognizable cell in the red blood cell line is called the rubriblast (also called pronormoblast), originating from the pluripotent stem hematopoietic cell. It is a large round cell (12 to 20 μ in diameter) and has a high nuclear-to-cytoplasm ratio of about 4:1. The nucleus is also large and round with a "lacy" fine chromatin that stains reddish-purple with Wright's stain. This chromatin material appears coarser than any of the white cell blast forms also found in the bone marrow. There may be up to two nucleoli visible in the nucleus as light blue staining circles. The cytoplasm has the distinctive deep blue coloration of blast forms, but there may be a reddish tint to it. Researchers, using radioactive iron, have shown that the iron needed for hemoglobin production enters the cell at this stage.

THE PRORUBRICYTE

Also called the basophilic normoblast, the second stage in the maturation of red cells shows a slightly smaller cell (10 to 16 μ in diameter) with a more abundant

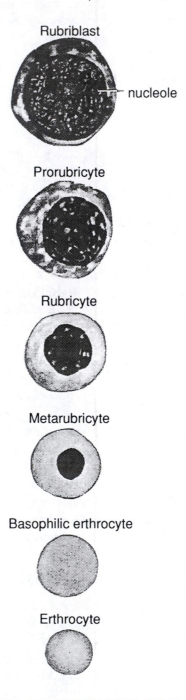

Rubriblast

nucleole

Prorubricyte

Rubricyte

Metarubricyte

Basophilic erthrocyte

Erthrocyte

fig. 6.1. Development of red blood cells. (From Marshall. *Fundamental Skills for the Clinical Laboratory Professional.* p. 314.)

cytoplasm. This cell is just about the size of an adult PMN. The nucleus, found in the center of the cell, shows a more clumped chromatin. There is an absence of nucleoli at this stage, helping to determine which of the two early cells are seen. The cytoplasm is deep blue in color. Hemoglobin production begins during this stage of development. There are also a few small masses of clumped chromatin located along the rim of the nuclear membrane.

THE RUBRICYTE

Also called the polychromatic normoblast, the third cell in the **mitotic pool** (those cell capable of reproduction) is the rubricyte, smaller than an adult PMN (10 to 12 µ in diameter). The nuclear/cytoplasmic ratio has decreased to 1:1. This is the first cell to show the production of hemoglobin because the cytoplasm is light gray. The chromatin in the nucleus continues to clump together, yielding a much darker staining nuclear mass. This cell may be mistaken for a lymphocyte. Look for the "company it keeps" to help determine its cell line.

THE METARUBRICYTE

Also called the orthochromic normoblast, the fourth cell in the development of red cells is a much smaller cell than those previously discussed, being 8 to 10 µ in diameter. The nucleus is described as **pyknotic** (dense compacted chromatin) and is very small and round in the center of the cell. It occupies only about one fourth the size of the cell. In late stages it will fragment and become eccentrically

E X E R C I S E **IDENTIFICATION OF MATURING RED BLOOD CELLS**

Purpose: Identifying maturing red blood cells in the bone marrow can familiarize the laboratory scientist with forms that can be found in the peripheral circulation in certain disease states.

Equipment Needed: Bone marrow smears provided by the instructor.

Procedure:
1. Using the oil immersion lens, bring the bone marrow smear into focus. Focus first on low power.
2. Locate an area that is associated with maturing red blood cells.
3. Try to locate as many examples of maturing red blood cells as possible.
4. Draw what you see. Be sure to check with the instructor about your cell identification.

Note: Color plates in a hematology reference textbook can be very helpful in determining the subtle differences in the maturing cells.

located near the plasma membrane. The nucleus will be extruded from this cell at the end of this stage. The cytoplasm is pink or orange-pink, with only a tinge of blue.

RETICULOCYTES

Referred to in Figure 6.1 as the basophilic erythrocyte, this cell is the first of the red cell line normally found in the peripheral circulation. Reticulocytes are actually young erythrocytes containing some residual RNA (in the form of ribosomes) and mitochondria in the cytoplasm. As long as ribosomes are present, heme production continues. During normal cell production, the number of reticulocytes in the marrow equals the number in circulation.

Staining the Reticulocyte Smear

In the blood smear, reticulocytes cells can take on a bluish color with Wright's stain, referred to as **polychromatophilia**. This cell stays in the bone marrow for about 2 days after the loss of the nucleus. It takes about a day in peripheral circulation for the reticulocytes to become mature erythrocytes.

The immaturity of the reticulocyte is seen by staining basophilic substance that remains in the cytoplasm of the red blood cell, disappearing after a day or two. This substance can be stained by mixing blood with new methylene blue N or brilliant cresyl blue stain. The number of cells showing a network of fibers within the cytoplasm gives the physician information about the health and productivity of the patient's bone marrow. This test can be used in following the course of treatment for anemia.

The reticulocyte count is more time-consuming than difficult. The laboratory scientist must count a total of 1000 red cells, distinguishing between those with and those without the fibrous reticulum. Exercise 58 illustrates staining of reticulocytes.

Errors Associated with the Reticulocyte Count

There are several possible sources of error when performing the reticulocyte count. The filtering of the stain is essential because precipitated stain can make erythrocytes look like reticulocytes. Moisture in erythrocytes left over from poor drying of the slides may look like reticulocytes. Using the fine adjustment should eliminate this problem. Reticulocytes will retain their stained round areas, whereas water artifacts are lost as the focus is adjusted.

Other erythrocyte inclusions are sometimes mistaken for reticulocytes. Howell-Jolly bodies are seen as one or two deeply purple dots in the cytoplasm with no reticulum (fine connecting lines). Heinz bodies are seen at the edge of the erythrocyte and stain blue-green. Pappenheimer bodies are purple-staining mitochondria, ribosomes, and iron deposits that appear in small clusters.

Some Conditions That Can Show an Increase in the Reticulocyte Count:

Hereditary spherocytic anemia	Blood loss
Sickle cell anemia	Hemolytic anemia
Thalassemia major	Paroxysmal nocturnal hemoglobinuria
Erythroblastosis fetalis	Treatment of pernicious anemia

E X E R C I S E `58` **STAINING THE RETICULOCYTE SMEAR**

SAFETY TECHNIQUE: WEAR GLOVES AND USE SHARPS CONTAINER FOR GLASS.

Purpose: The reticulocyte smear is observed to determine the production of red blood cells by counting reticulated cells on a stained blood smear.

Equipment Needed: Latex gloves, EDTA blood sample, new methylene blue N solution (or brilliant cresyl blue), glass slides, small test tube, Pasteur pipette, microscope, filter paper and funnel, biohazard container.

Procedure:
1. Mix the sample of EDTA blood to be tested by inversion of the vacuum tube or by a rotating mixer.
2. While the blood is mixing, filter about 0.5 ml of a 1% solution of new methylene blue N stain (or brilliant cresyl blue) into a small test tube.
3. Using a Pasteur pipette, extract approximately 4 to 5 drops of the filtered stain and place it in a small test tube. This tube will act as the mixing tube.
4. Add to the filtered stain 3 drops of EDTA blood (well mixed). Mix the two together by holding the test tube with one hand and tapping along the side of the tube with the other.
5. Allow to stand for at least 5 minutes and then remix.
6. Extract a drop of the mixture and place it on a glass slide. Using another slide, smear the mixture across the slide in the same manner that differential slides are prepared.
7. Allow to air dry. The slide will be greenish in color.
8. Place on a microscope stage and bring the slide into focus using low power. Then switch to oil (with a drop of oil) in the same manner used with viewing the differential slide.
9. Ask your instructor to verify that the stain has been properly performed.

Some Conditions That Can Show a Decrease in the Reticulocyte Count:

Aplastic anemia	Pernicious anemia
Decreased erythropoiesis	Chemotherapy or radiation
Inducing hypoproliferation	

Absolute Reticulocyte Count

The absolute reticulocyte count provides a comparable basis for following the progression of anemia and its treatment. This count expresses the number of

E X E R C I S E   **59**   **COUNTING RETICULOCYTES**

Purpose: Reticulocytes are counted to demonstrate the production rate of erythrocytes.

Equipment Needed: New methylene blue stained smear (see Exercise 58).

Procedure:
1. Place a drop of immersion oil on the thin area of the slide.
2. Using the oil immersion objective (100X), bring the field into focus. Focus on low power first.
3. Find the area of the smear where the red cells are just touching each other—the feathered area.
4. Using the fine adjustment, move into and just out of focus. Look for red cells that have dark round spots and/or filaments connecting stained areas. These are the reticulocytes.
5. The reticulocytes must be counted along with normal red cells to 1000 cells. Five hundred can be counted on two different smears. A special eyepiece with a crossline dividing the field of vision into four quadrants is available. It is placed in the ocular. The larger of the two areas is nine times the area of the smaller area. Reticulocytes are counted in the larger area, and red cells are counted in the smaller area.

CALCULATIONS: Using the crossline disc or no disc in the counting, 1000 red blood cells are counted. Example: 7 reticulocytes are counted within the 1000 count. The calculation and the reported percentage would be achieved using this formula:

$$\frac{7 \text{ reticulocytes counted}}{1000 \text{ red cells counted, including reticulocytes}} \times 100 = 0.7\%$$

NORMAL VALUES: 2.5% to 6.5% newborns (decreasing to adult range by second week)
0.5% to 1.5% adult range

reticulocytes in 1 cu mm of whole blood; it is not an RBC percentage. The normal value is 60,000/cu mm. This value is obtained by the following formula:

$$\frac{\text{Reticulocyte count (\%)}}{100} \times \text{RBC count (per } \mu l)$$

Example:
$$\frac{1.5\% \times 4.0 \text{ million/cu mm}}{100} = 60,000/\text{cu mm}$$

Correcting the Reticulocyte Count for Anemia

Anemia is a condition in which the production of red blood cells is decreased, their ability to carry oxygen is hindered, or they are being destroyed or lost faster than they can be produced. The reticulocyte count needs to be corrected to account for variations in the erythrocyte quantity present.

THE MATURE ERYTHROCYTE

The typical erythrocyte is a small biconcave disc with a volume of 80 to 100 fl (**femtoliter**). It measures about 6.8 to 7.5 μ in diameter. It stains pink using Wright's stain because of the quantities of hemoglobin that are acidophilic. The mature red blood cell has lost its residual RNA, mitochondria, and some enzymes. This cell is incapable of synthesizing proteins or lipids and has a limited life span of about 120 days.

THE ERYTHROCYTE MEMBRANE

The erythrocyte membrane is essential for red cell function and survival. If the membrane is defective either by inherited or acquired abnormalities, severe ane-

---

E X E R C I S E   60   CORRECTING THE RETICULOCYTE COUNT

SAFETY TECHNIQUE: NONE.

Purpose: Based on the normal hematocrit values of men and women, the reticulocyte count can be corrected for the degree of anemia present, using the following formula:

$$\text{Corrected reticulocyte count (\%)} = \text{reticulocyte count (\%)} \times \frac{\text{patient hematocrit}}{\text{normal hematocrit*}}$$

Procedure:

1. Calculate the corrected reticulocyte count, given the following:
   Adult male hematocrit is 35% (0.35 L/L)
   Normal adult male hematocrit value is 45% (0.45 L/L)
   Uncorrected reticulocyte count = 3.5%

   $$\text{Corrected reticulocyte} = 3.5\% \times \frac{0.35 \text{ L/L}}{0.45 \text{ L/L}}$$

   Corrected reticulocyte count = 2.7%, multiplying the result by 100 to convert to a percentage.

2. Calculate on your own: A female patient has an uncorrected reticulocyte count of 3.2%. Her hematocrit is 29%, with the normal female hematocrit being 42% for women.

*Normal hematocrit is calculated differently for men and women.

E X E R C I S E ▮61▮ IDENTIFICATION OF THE ERYTHROCYTE

SAFETY TECHNIQUE: WEAR GLOVES.

Purpose: The erythrocyte is the most numerous cell in the differential smear. The laboratory scientist must be able to recognize abnormalities of these abundant cells.

Equipment Needed: Blood smears created by the student and appropriately stained with Wright's stain.

Procedure:
1. Bring the blood smear into focus using the oil immersion lens (100X) after first focusing on low power.
2. Locate the thin portion of the smear where the red cells are just about touching each other.
3. Make a drawing of several erythrocytes. Notice that the cells can vary in size and shape. Try to include in the drawing any variations in the cells in the field of vision.

mias can result. The membrane must be flexible so that the red blood cell can squeeze through the small capillaries of the spleen. This flexibility must also be accompanied by a fluidity within the red blood cell, composed mainly of hemoglobin (Figure 6.2). Any change in membrane flexibility or cytoplasmic fluidity results in the cells becoming trapped in the spleen and/or being destroyed by macrophages.

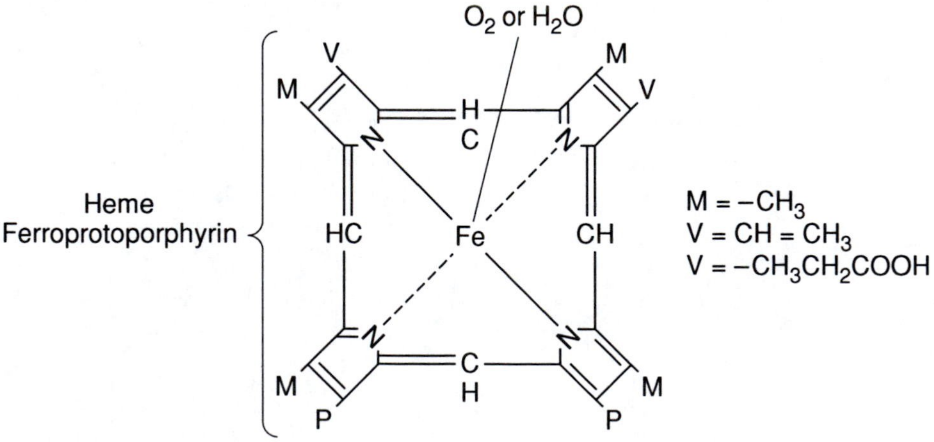

$$M = -CH_3$$
$$V = CH = CH_3$$
$$V = -CH_3CH_2COOH$$

fig. 6.2. Structure of hemoglobin. (From Marshall. *Fundamental Skills for the Clinical Laboratory Professional.* p. 320.)

The red blood cell membrane is a bilayer of phospholipids, proteins, and carbohydrates (49% proteins, 43% lipids, and 8% carbohydrates). Any defect in the membrane can alter all functions and lead to premature death of the cell.

MORPHOLOGIC ERYTHROCYTIC ABNORMALITIES

Red cell abnormalities can cause **anisocytosis,** a variation in size of the red blood cell. Cells that are smaller than the normal red cell (6.8 to 7.5 μ in diameter) are called **microcytic.** Cells averaging 8.2 μ in diameter are called **macrocytes.** The size variations are used in the morphologic classification of some anemias.

Conditions that cause these changes in size have a physiologic basis. Macrocytes are the result of either a defect in the nucleus, caused by a deficiency of vitamin B$_{12}$ or folate, or by an increased synthesis of hemoglobin while the cell was in the mitotic pool. This causes the cells to not only appear larger than normal, but to take on a bluish coloration (basophilia) and be slightly **hypochromic** on the smear.

Microcytosis is caused by a decrease in hemoglobin production, possibly the result of iron deficiency, impaired globulin synthesis, or an abnormality in the synthesis of heme. Examples of disorders with microcytosis are iron-deficiency anemia and the thalassemias. Variations in the disc shape of an erythrocyte represent a change in the contents of the cell or its membrane. These variations in erythrocyte shape are called **poikilocytosis.** As with anisocytosis, poikilocytosis is a general term; when a more appropriate term can be used, it should be. A partial list of red blood cell shape variations follows.

Acanthocyte: This is a cell with multiple spines projecting from the membrane. These cells are found in cirrhosis of the liver with associated hemolytic anemia, in neonatal hepatitis, and after splenectomy.

Burr cell: Also called an echinocyte, this cell has blunt projections, unlike the pointed projections of acanthocytes. The Burr cell is seen in a number of anemias, gastric and peptic ulcers, gastric carcinoma, uremia, and dehydration (Figure 6.3).

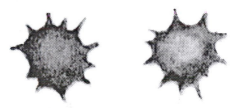

fig. 6.3. Burr cells. (From Marshall. *Fundamental Skills for the Clinical Laboratory Professional.* p. 360.)

Dacryocyte: This cell is also called a teardrop cell because of its pointed end with the other side being rounded, like a tear or a pear. The cell obtains this shape when the spleen "bites" out inclusions. It is seen in megaloblastic anemia, thalassemia, some cancers, and myeloid metaplasia.

Drepanocyte: This cell is also called a *sickle cell* because of its distinctive shape (Figure 6.4). Individuals with sickle cell anemia will have these cells. A low oxygen concentration and pressure in the peripheral blood causes sickling of the cells. This cell is diagnostic for sickle cell anemia.

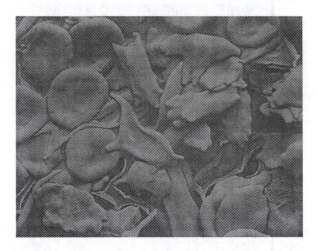

fig. 6.4. Sickled red blood cells. (Courtesy of Philips Electronic Instruments Company.)

Elliptocyte: This cell shape can be inherited, with some patients having few problems and others having serious anemia. It can also be seen in iron-deficiency and certain hemolytic anemias (Figure 6.5).

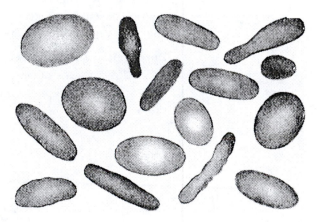

fig. 6.5. Elliptocytes. (From Marshall. *Fundamental Skills for the Clinical Laboratory Professional.* p. 339.)

Leptocyte: These cells are also known as target cells, Mexican hat cells, and codocytes. The central portion is dark, like the periphery. The cell has a target appearance. They are seen in thalassemia, some hemoglobinopathies, hepatic disorders, and iron-deficiency anemia.

Schistocyte: Also called a schizocyte, helmet cell, bite cell, or red cell fragment to reflect this cell's shape, this is an important red blood cell to identify. This cell can appear in the condition known as disseminated intravascular coagulation (DIC), in which a patient's body initiates clotting mechanisms throughout the body. As red cells pass through the blood vessels of a patient with DIC, they may encounter strands of fibrin and be sliced in half. This is an extremely dangerous condition (to be discussed further in Unit 8), and evidence of DIC should be reported to a physician immediately. This cell can also be seen in burn patients and microangiopathic hemolytic anemia as well.

E X E R C I S E 62 **IDENTIFICATION OF SCHISTOCYTES (SCHIZOCYTES)**

Purpose: Schistocytes are characterized by their distinctive shapes. Identification of these cells can aid the physician in quickly diagnosing disseminated intravascular coagulation (DIC).

Equipment Needed: Blood smears provided by the instructor.

Procedure:
1. Using the oil immersion lens (100X), bring the blood smear into low power focus first.
2. Locate the thin area of the smear.
3. Locate cells that appear to be schistocytes. Verify your findings with your instructor.
4. Draw these cells.

Spherocytes: These cells are no longer biconcave, assuming a round shape. They appear as if the red blood cell has too much hemoglobin. Spherocytes (Figure 6.6) are usually found in an inherited abnormality, such as hereditary spherocytic anemia. They can also be seen in autoimmune hemolytic anemia, ABO hemolytic disease of the newborn, and acquired hemolytic anemias.

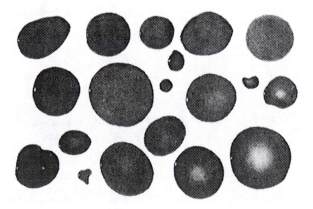

fig. 6.6. Spherocytes. (From Marshall. *Fundamental Skills for the Clinical Laboratory Professional.* p. 338.)

Stomatocyte: This is an abnormal red blood cell (Figure 6.7) with a central area shaped like a mouth, more of a slit than a circle. This cell is associated with a hemolytic anemia, as well as acute alcoholism and alcoholic cirrhosis.

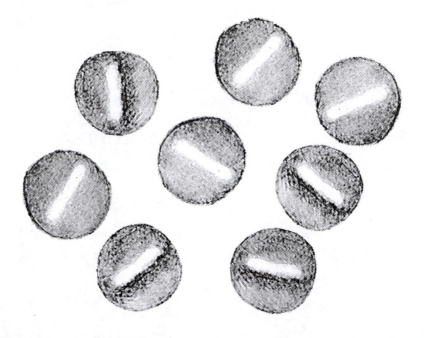

fig. 6.7. Stomatocytes. (From Marshall. *Fundamental Skills for the Clinical Laboratory Professional.* p. 340.)

E X E R C I S E **63** **IDENTIFICATION OF ABNORMAL RED BLOOD CELLS**

Purpose: Accurate identification of abnormal red blood cell morphology gives the physician diagnostic information.

Equipment Needed: Blood smears provided by the instructor.

Procedure:
1. Using the oil immersion lens (100X), bring the blood smear into focus.
2. Locate the thin area of the smear.
3. Locate red blood cells that are normal in shape. You may want to view several slides to be able to see a wide variation in shape.
4. Locate abnormal red blood cells and attempt to name them. Check with your instructor if you are not sure of the identifications. It is very helpful to use color plates of abnormal red blood cells to help in the identification. These can be found in hematology reference textbooks.
5. Make drawings of these cells.

RED BLOOD CELL DESTRUCTION

The destruction of red cells normally takes place because of old age, since these cells are not able to reproduce. With aging, enzyme activity begins to slow down and red blood cells lose the ability to maintain their shape. Most of the red blood cells are removed from circulation by the liver, spleen, and bone marrow. A small number are destroyed by white cells in circulation, releasing some hemoglobin.

ERYTHROCYTE INCLUSIONS

Red cells that have deposits of RNA, precipitated nuclear material, or parasites are said to have inclusions. Sometimes special stains must be used to locate and define the inclusions. Stains such as new methylene blue or brilliant cresyl blue are used to demonstrate the presence of RNA. These stains are called supravital stains, meaning that cells are stained while living. Those that demonstrate the presence of DNA are called Feulgen stains. Some inclusions can be demonstrated with Wright's or crystal violet stains (also a supravital stain).

Basophilic stippling: This name is given to inclusions in erythrocytes appearing as fine or coarse gray-black granules. They are usually evenly distributed and of uniform size. Cells with basophilic stippling are generally young cells in which normal reticulocyte basophilia has been altered. These are seen in many anemias, in heavy metal poisoning, especially lead poisoning, and in thalassemias.

Cabot rings: A small ring shape or looped figure is seen in red blood cells. These may correspond to the nuclear remnants or histone synthesis. They are seen in lead poisoning and pernicious anemia. However, the exact origin of these rings is still uncertain.

Heinz bodies: These are small round inclusions that stain deep purple with crystal violet stain. They are usually located near the edge of the erythrocyte. They are precipitated denatured hemoglobin and are associated with hemolytic anemias, G6PD deficiency, and some hemoglobinopathies. The Wright's stain will not show these inclusions.

Howell-Jolly bodies: These are seen as single or double dots on the red cell. They are nuclear remnants composed of DNA and are thought to indicate abnormal erythropoiesis. They are present when the spleen cannot remove unwanted nuclear debris. They are seen in hemolytic and pernicious anemias as well as when damage to the spleen is present.

Pappenheimer bodies: These are also called siderotic particles. When Wright's stain is used, Pappenheimer bodies are characterized by purple dots that are aggregates of ribosomes and/or mitochondria. Pappenheimer bodies are seen in hemolytic anemias, iron-loading anemias, and hyposplenism.

PARASITIC INCLUSIONS

Several parasites are found in human blood, including protozoa (one-celled microscopic organisms) and parasitic worms. Red blood cells can be invaded by

EXERCISE 64 IDENTIFICATION OF ERYTHROCYTE INCLUSIONS

Purpose: Proper identification of red blood cell inclusions can give the physician important information about disease processes.

Equipment Needed: Blood smears provided by the instructor.

Procedure:
1. Using the oil immersion lens (100X), bring the blood smear into focus, using low power first.
2. Locate the thin area of the smear.
3. Locate cells that have inclusions. A hematology reference textbook with color plates of red blood cell inclusions would be helpful for accurate identification.
4. Consult your instructor for verification of what you see.
5. You may have to view several slides (or the instructor may set up several microscopes with different inclusions to be viewed).
6. Draw what you see.

parasites, especially a species of protozoans known as malarial parasites, belonging to the Coccidia group of protozoans.

Malarial parasites are called **plasmodium** species, of which there are four separate species. Plasmodium are the parasites usually discussed in hematology because they are found in red cells. The four species are:

- *Plasmodium vivax* (the most common species)
- *Plasmodium falciparum*
- *Plasmodium malariae*
- *Plasmodium ovale*

These four species are all called malaria and can be found in different stages in their life cycles in the red cells.

The *gametocyte* stage, which is formed in the human host, is ingested by the **vector** insect, the Anopheles mosquito. This stage has two developing gametes, microgametes and macrogametes, that fuse to form a *zygote*. This zygote constricts and is called the *oocyst*. The oocyst then produces many fine threadlike **sporozoites**. The sporozoites enter the salivary glands of the mosquito, transferring to a host through the mosquito's bite. The development of the sporozoites depends on the outside temperature and can take between 8 and 35 days.

In the human, the sporozoite enters the bloodstream through a mosquito bite. Within 40 minutes, it has entered the liver to undergo asexual reproduction. Individual parasites increase, becoming thousands of **merozoites**. The liver cells rupture, and the merozoites enter circulation to infect red blood cells. Each red cell infected produces from four to thirty-six new parasites. The red cell ruptures, causing chills followed by a fever at regular intervals. These cyclical fevers help the physician diagnosis malaria.

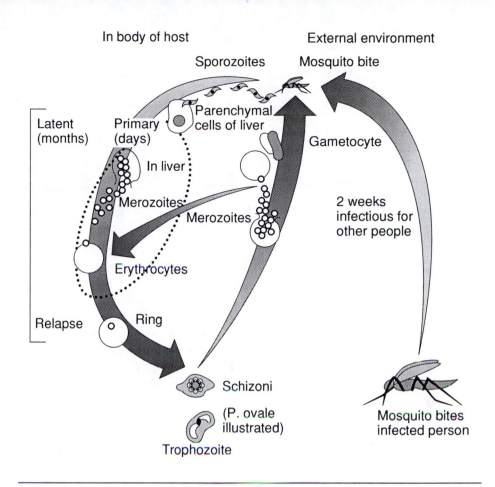

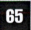

fig. 6.8. *Plasmodium* life cycle. (From Marshall. *Fundamental Skills for the Clinical Laboratory Professional.* p. 610.)

The most common form of malaria is *Plasmodium vivax*. It is seen in red cells as a ring form called a **trophozoite**. There is usually a blue ring with a red dot associated with it. It is advisable to make both thick and thin smears (Exercise 65) if malaria is suspected. The thick smear is used to look for the trophozoites, though they may appear distorted. Gametocytes of *P. vivax, P. ovale,* and *P. malariae* are very similar.

E X E R C I S E 🔳65 **PREPARING THICK AND THIN MALARIA BLOOD SMEARS**

SAFETY TECHNIQUE: WEAR GLOVES.

Purpose: Properly stained malaria blood smears are essential for proper species identification of malaria.

Equipment Needed: Field's rapid stain and Leishman stain (prepared by instructor), blood smears with malarial parasites, tap water, methyl alcohol, stain rack, tweezers, latex gloves, biohazard container, disinfectant.

EXERCISE  PREPARING THICK AND THIN MALARIA
BLOOD SMEARS *(continued)*

Procedure for Thick Film:
1. Wash hands thoroughly and put on latex gloves.
2. Thick blood smear is made by placing a medium-size drop of blood on a clean slide and spreading it with another slide until it covers an area of about 2 cm in diameter. It is then allowed to dry (you may not have malarial blood available for this procedure).
3. Immerse dried, unfixed blood smear for 1 to 3 seconds in solution 1 of Field's rapid stain.
4. Remove and rinse immediately for about 5 seconds in tap water until no more stain comes from the film.
5. Immerse in solution 2 for 2 seconds.
6. Rinse for 2 to 3 seconds in tap water. Let stand to drain and dry.

Thin Film:
1. Thin films can be made like a regular differential blood smear. You may not have malarial blood available and will be provided with a ready-made smear.
2. Fix thin films by adding a few drops of methyl alcohol. Leave for a few seconds.
3. Pour off alcohol and, before films dry, apply diluted Leishman stain.
4. Stain for 30 minutes.
5. Hold the slide under a steady stream of water for approximately 15 seconds.
6. Allow stains to drain and dry before examining.
7. Dispose properly of all biohazardous waste products. Disinfect area where contamination might have occurred.

Note: Your instructor may want to use alternate methods of staining. There are several stains that can be used for this purpose.

ADDITIONAL ERYTHROCYTE ABNORMALITIES

Rouleau Formation: This formation, discussed in Unit 5 in connection with multiple myeloma (see Exercise 55), is described as red blood cells appearing as "stacked coins." Red blood cells lining up like this can be seen in thick portions of blood smears. If rouleau is found in thin portions, it is abnormal and should be reported. It can be caused by an increase in plasma globulin, as in multiple myeloma.

Agglutination: Red blood cells sticking together can be caused by incompatible blood being given during a transfusion. This phenomenon is caused by antibodies reacting with antigens. This will be seen in all areas of the smear. A

EXERCISE 66 IDENTIFICATION OF MALARIAL PARASITES

Purpose: The identification of malarial parasites requires fresh blood specimens, well-stained smears, and experienced laboratory scientists to make proper identifications.

Equipment needed: Blood smears provided by instructor, color plates from laboratory reference textbooks.

Procedure:

1. After first focusing on low power, focus the microscope under oil immersion, then identify the malarial parasites provided by your instructor. Proper identification takes much practice!
2. Answer the following questions on a separate piece of paper:
   - Which malaria is most deadly?
   - Which malaria is the most widespread?
   - How much malaria is reported in your area?
   - What is being done worldwide to eliminate malaria?

blood smear should be made if a transfusion reaction is suspected. Incompatible blood transfusions are potentially lethal to the patient if not caught immediately. Agglutination can also be seen in patients with cold agglutinins when blood is allowed to cool before the blood smear is made. The hematologist should always watch for red blood cell agglutination.

HEMOGLOBIN

The hemoglobin level is a determination of the amount of oxygen-carrying capability of the red blood cells. This test is often abbreviated on laboratory report forms as *Hb* or *Hgb*. It is the initial test to determine if an anemic condition exists. The hemoglobin value varies with age, sex, and geographic location. The highest normal value is at birth, but lowers within the first week. Females have lower values than males because of their smaller mass size, and pregnant females can have a lower value during the second and third trimesters. Both male and female levels lower at about age 65 years. To be able to understand what the results mean, a brief explanation of the synthesis of hemoglobin is necessary.

SYNTHESIS OF HEMOGLOBIN

The synthesis of hemoglobin requires the presence of iron, protoporphyrin IX (roman numerals are used with protoporphyrins), amino acids, RNA, and enzymes. In the synthesis, enzymes process iron and protoporphyrin to form a complex called heme. The amino acids, RNA, and enzymes together make the

EXERCISE **67** **ERYTHROCYTE AGGLUTINATION CAUSED BY INCOMPATIBLE BLOOD GROUPS**

SAFETY TECHNIQUE: WEAR GLOVES.

Purpose: Agglutination of red blood cells can be caused by incompatible blood groups being mixed together.

Equipment Needed: Two tubes of EDTA blood (different blood types), Wright's stain, test tube, and slides.

Procedure:

1. Take 5 drops of blood from one anticoagulated blood tube and place it in the test tube.
2. Take 5 drops of blood from the second tube and place it in the same test tube.
3. Mix and allow to stand for 5 minutes.
4. Make several blood smears.
5. Stain smears with Wright's stain.
6. After focusing on low power, use the oil immersion lens (100X) and bring the blood smear into focus.
7. Locate the thin area of the smear.
8. Locate the agglutination formation and make a drawing of it.
9. Dispose properly of all biohazardous waste products.

carrier molecules called globin, which unite with the heme to form hemoglobin. As the amount of hemoglobin increases within the cell, the amount of RNA decreases. This is why the color of the cytoplasm changes from blue to pink during maturation. This process takes about 1 week to complete. Each red cell produces about 280 million molecules of hemoglobin, with the rest of the cell being filled with water (see Figure 6.2).

The amino acid chains are of four types: alpha, beta, delta, and gamma. These amino acid chains are found as identical pairs. The alpha chains consist of 141 amino acids. The beta chains consists of 146 amino acids. These two types of hemoglobin chains constitute about 95% of the total adult hemoglobin and are called hemoglobin A.

When hemoglobin is carrying oxygen, it is bright red in color and is called oxyhemoglobin. When it is carrying carbon dioxide (most of which is carried in the plasma), it is called reduced hemoglobin. It is the presence of the iron in the ferrous state (Fe^{++}) that forms a temporary bond with oxygen to transport it to the body tissues. If the ferrous iron is oxidized, it forms a ferric iron (Fe^{+++}), and is then called methemoglobin. Normal blood contains 0.1% methemoglobin.

It is important to know the difference between relative and absolute amounts of hemoglobin. Relative concentration is the amount of hemoglobin in relationship to the volume of plasma. If the plasma volume increases, the hemoglobin concentration decreases. Absolute concentration is the total hemoglobin mass independent of the plasma volume. If the plasma volume increases, the hemoglobin concentration remains constant. This is helpful in dealing with anemias.

Changes in altitude change the hemoglobin because there is a physiologic adjustment of the body to deal with the lower oxygen levels.

HEMOGLOBIN TESTING

Several methods have been used to determine the concentration of hemoglobin within a given amount of blood. Today, hemoglobin results are automatically read in sophisticated cell counters by spectrophotometers.

Several methods used in the past (and some still in use today as back-up methods) are listed below.

- The *Tallqvist* and the *Dare's* methods were seriously inaccurate in their results because both methods require a color value judgment on the part of the laboratory scientist.
- The *acid hematin* method (called the Sahli-Hellige procedure) required the mixing of a sample of blood with hydrochloric acid to produce a brownish colored solution, which was then compared with a standard. This method was slightly inaccurate.
- The *alkali hematin* method (called the Haden-Hausser procedure) required that a sodium hydroxide solution be added to a blood sample and then boiled, yielding a greenish- to bluish-colored solution which was compared with a standard. This method was generally considered accurate, but could not be used with infant hemoglobin.
- The *cyanomethemoglobin* method requires the mixing of a cyanide solution called Drabkin's reagent to a sample of blood. The oxidized result is read in a spectrophotometer.

HEMATOCRIT

The hematocrit is a test to determine the ratio between the formed elements and the plasma after centrifugation. Recall that blood consists of a cellular portion, usually called the formed elements, and a liquid portion called the plasma. This test is abbreviated as *Hct* and is also called the *packed cell volume*. It is commonly reported as a percent, but some prefer to report the results as Liter/Liter.

The ranges of normal hematocrit reading for a large population are listed in Table 6.1.

Table 6.1. Hematocrit Normals

Adult males	0.40–0.54 L/L
Adult females	0.37–0.47 L/L
Infants	0.28–0.45 L/L
Newborns	0.50–0.70 L/L

E X E R C I S E  **IDENTIFICATION OF BLOOD COMPONENTS**

SAFETY TECHNIQUE: WEAR GLOVES.

Purpose: Gravity will position heavy objects at the bottom of a container and less dense objects above.

Equipment Needed: Anticoagulated blood, test tube rack, timer, biohazard container.

Procedure:
1. Obtain an anticoagulated blood sample and place it in the test tube rack.
2. Let it stand for a period of 4 hours.
3. Make an observation of the blood tube after the allotted time and make a drawing of the results.
4. Determine the ratio of cells to plasma. This is a simplified hematocrit test.
5. Observe the buffy coat layer, where the white blood cells and platelets fall between the plasma and red blood cells.
6. Dispose of all biohazardous wastes properly.

E X E R C I S E  **THE MANUAL HEMATOCRIT**

SAFETY TECHNIQUE: WEAR GLOVES.

Purpose: The ratio of cells and plasma is found by centrifuging a capillary tube and measuring the result.

Equipment Needed: Anticoagulated blood, capillary tubes, microhematocrit centrifuge with timer, microhematocrit reader, sealing clay, biohazard container.

Procedure:
1. Wearing gloves, fill the capillary tube two-thirds full with anticoagulated blood.
2. Place one end of the capillary tube into clay to close off one end.
3. Place capillary tube into a microhematocrit centrifuge with the sealed end toward the perimeter. It is not necessary to balance the capillary tube.
4. Replace the cover and screw it down tightly.

E X E R C I S E　**69**　**THE MANUAL HEMATOCRIT** *(continued)*

5. Set the timer to 5 minutes. The centrifuge should start moving. To ensure proper rpm, the centrifuge should be calibrated regularly.
6. When the centrifuge shuts off, be sure to let it come to a full stop before opening the top.
7. Remove the tube. Using a microhematocrit reader, place the sealed end so that the blood touches the straight line. This is the base line from which the ratio is calculated.
8. Bring the curved line down until it intersects the plasma.
   Note: various models of readers are available.
9. Holding the side of the numerical readings, turn them until the curved line (above) intersects the packed red cell mass (below the buffy coat).
10. Look down to the numerical wheel and read off the hematocrit value.
11. Report results as a percent.
12. Dispose of all biohazardous waste properly.

POSSIBLE ERRORS IN HEMATOCRIT VALUES

Hematocrit results, like hemoglobin determinations, can change with geographical location. When fluids are lost from the body in conditions such as relative polycythemia, vomiting, diarrhea, heavy sweating, or severe burns, the hematocrit and hemoglobin values are artificially increased due to the decrease in plasma fluids.

The gain of fluids in the body during the premenstrual period, pregnancy, or heavy liquid intake can falsely decrease the hematocrit and hemoglobin. Other conditions that falsely increase the hematocrit include hyperglycemia and hypernatremia (high sodium levels). Other errors in the hematocrit values can include the following:

- If the test is performed immediately after an episode of hemorrhage, the results will yield a false high result.
- If there is too much anticoagulant in drawing the blood, the results will yield a false low result due to the shrinking of red blood cells.
- If the blood is not mixed enough before performing the test, it will yield either a false high or low result, depending on where the sample is taken. Blood must be thoroughly mixed before using.
- Failure to centrifuge properly can cause erroneous results.
- Leakage of blood from the microcapillary tube can skew results. Observe the centrifuge each time it is used to see if any blood is found on the inside of the centrifuge.

ERYTHROCYTE SEDIMENTATION RATE (ESR)

The erythrocyte sedimentation rate is a test to determine the rate of fall of the red cells in a glass tube over a period of 1 hour. The fall of these cells is measured in millimeters and is dependent upon many variables. These variables include an increase in body fluids as in pregnancy, the production of excess proteins as in multiple myeloma or an inflammatory reaction, or a decrease in the red cell mass as seen in hemolytic anemia.

The sedimentation rate is partly governed by the length and diameter of the glass tube used in the test. Normal values vary according to procedure utilized. The ESR is not specific for any particular disease but is used as one test in a battery of tests for diagnosis.

EXERCISE 70 THE WESTERGREN ERYTHROCYTE SEDIMENTATION RATE

SAFETY TECHNIQUE: WEAR GLOVES.

Purpose: Same as for Wintrobe method.

Equipment Needed: EDTA blood, Westergren tubes, a Westergren tube rack, automatic pipettor, timer, soft laboratory tissues, normal saline to change volume (use 4:1 ratio of 2 ml blood and 0.5 ml saline), biohazardous waste container.

Procedure:
1. Mix the blood sample until needed, then dilute.
2. Wearing gloves and using an automatic pipettor, draw the blood into the Westergren tube, slightly overfilling it.
3. Use the index finger to cover the top of the Westergren tube. Bring the tube to eye level. Gently allow the blood meniscus to drop to the zero mark.
4. Wipe off any excess blood with a soft laboratory tissue.
5. Place the Westergren tube into the rack and make sure it is vertical.
6. Set the timer for 1 hour.
7. In 1 hour, read the level of the meniscus of the blood in the tube. Record the results, reporting results in millimeters per hour.
8. Properly dispose of all biohazardous materials.
   Normal Values: Males   0 to 15 mm/hr
                   Females   0 to 20 mm/hr

SOME SOURCES OF ERROR WHEN PERFORMING THE ESR

- Excessive anticoagulant decreases the rate of blood cell settling.
- Partially clotted blood decreases the rate of settling. The specimen must be properly mixed before performing the ESR.
- Blood must be fresh. For the Wintrobe method, the test should be performed within 1 hour. For the Westergren method, the test should be performed within 2 hours.
- Air bubbles in the tube can interfere with accurate results.
- If the ESR tube is not completely vertical, accurate results will not be obtained.

SOME CONDITIONS THAT CAN HAVE A HIGH ESR

Rheumatic fever	Pregnancy
Pneumonia	Nephritis
Cancer	Multiple myeloma
Syphilis	Tuberculosis
Rouleau formation	Sickle cell anemia
Anemia	Leukemia
Menstruation	Nephrosis
Thalassemia	

RED BLOOD CELL INDICES

The red cell indices are calculations using the red blood cell count, hemoglobin, and hematocrit values to help classify red blood cells as to size and hemoglobin content. It is useful when determining if an anemia exists and to identify the type of anemia. There are three calculations included in this group: the *mean corpuscular volume (MCV)*, the *mean corpuscular hemoglobin (MCH)*, and the *mean corpuscular hemoglobin concentration (MCHC)*. Another parameter that is also included on hematology analyzers is the red blood cell distribution width (RDW).

To calculate the indices you must have the red blood cell count and the hemoglobin and the hematocrit values. For the *MCV*, which indicates the average volume of individual red cells in femtoliters (fl = 1×10^{-15} or 1 quadrillionth of a liter), you would divide the hematocrit by the red blood cell count.

$$MCV = \frac{Hct\ ([\%] \times 10)}{RBC\ (in\ millions/cu\ mm)}$$

The MCV is reported in the following units: $fl(\mu^3)$.

Using the MCV, cells are classified as normocytic (80 to 100 fl), microcytic (less than 80 fl), and macrocytic (greater than 100 fl). The above example (93 fl) is within the normocytic classification.

The *MCH* is a measurement of the average weight of hemoglobin in a single red cell expressed in picograms (1×10^{-12}, or 1 trillionth of a gram). It is calculated by dividing the hemoglobin value times 10 by the RBC, as below:

$$MCH\ (pg) = \frac{Hb\ (g \times 100\ ml) \times 10}{RBC\ (millions/cu\ mm)}$$

The MCH is reported in picograms (pg).

The MCH for normocytic erythrocytes is between 27 and 31 pg; for macrocytic erythrocytes it is above 31 pg; for microcytic it is below 27 pg. The MCH should always correlate with the MCV and MCHC. Smaller cells should contain less hemoglobin molecules, and larger cells should contain more hemoglobin molecules.

The *MCHC* is a measurement of the average concentration of hemoglobin in grams in a deciliter (100 ml) of red cells. It is calculated by dividing the hemoglobin value by the hematocrit value as below:

$$\text{MCHC (g/dl)} = \frac{\text{Hb (g/100 ml)} \times 10}{\text{Hct ([\%]} \times 10)}$$

The MCHC is reported in the following units: g/liter.

The MCHC describes the erythrocytes as being either normochromic (31 to 36 g/dl) or hypochromic (values less than 31 g/dl). Cells with values greater than 36 g/dl are spherocytes (this was once called hyperchromic).

RDW

The **RDW** (red blood cell distribution width) is the coefficient of variation of the red blood cell volume distribution. This value is obtained directly from the histogram in automated cell counters. The normal value for the RDW is 11.5% to 14.5%. All abnormalities in the RDW at present have been found above 14.5%, indicating anisocytosis (a variation in the size of cells). This is seen in iron-deficiency anemia and vitamin B_{12} and folic acid deficiency. The more anemic the

---

E X E R C I S E   **CALCULATING RED BLOOD CELL INDICES**

Purpose: The student gains experience in manually calculating the three most commonly used RBC indices—the MCV, the MCH, and the MCHC.

Procedure:
1. Use the following values and the equations listed in the preceding section to calculate mean corpuscular volume (MCV), mean corpuscular hemoglobin (MCH), and mean corpuscular hemoglobin concentration (MCHC).
2. Hematocrit = 43%
   Red blood cell count = 4.7 million/cu mm
   Hemoglobin = 14.0 g/100 ml
3. Compare your answers to other students. Verify answers with the instructor. **Don't forget to report results in the proper units.**
4. Repeat calculations using the following values: Hematocrit = 37%, Hemoglobin = 12.2 g/100 ml, RBC = 4.1 million/cu mm.
5. Again, check your answers.

individual, the higher the RDW. To calculate the RDW, the standard deviation of the red cell size and the mean for the sample must be known. Divide the standard deviation by the mean and multiply by 100.

$$\text{RDW (\%)} = \frac{\text{SD}}{\text{mean}} \times 100$$

Today the indices and RDW are calculated by automated equipment, but you should know how to achieve these values. The hematocrit value is also a calculation with automated equipment.

SUMMARY

The erythrocyte (red blood cell), about 7 μ in diameter, is of vital importance in maintaining homeostasis. It carries oxygen to the cells and removes wastes for excretion. The maturation of the erythrocyte involves the elimination of the nucleus. This increases the area within the cell to carry oxygen. The most immature form of the red blood cell is the rubriblast, followed by the prorubricyte, the rubricyte, the metarubricyte, the reticulocyte, and finally the mature erythrocyte.

The reticulocyte is the first red blood cell to be found in the peripheral circulation. It is a young erythrocyte containing some residual RNA and mitochondria in the cytoplasm. Stained with Wright's stain, reticulocytes can take on a bluish color and can be counted. When their numbers increase, it can be concluded that increased production of red blood cells is taking place. The absolute reticulocyte count expresses the number of reticulocytes in 1 cu mm of blood. A reticulocyte count needs to be corrected when there are variations in the erythrocyte quantity present.

The mature erythrocyte can have defects of its membrane, as well as other morphologic abnormalities. Such abnormalities can include anisocytosis (variation in size), including microcytosis (smaller than normal) and macrocytosis (larger than normal). Cells can be hypochromic (less than normal color). Poikilocytosis (variation in shape) produces many different types of cells, including acanthocytes, burr cells, dacryocytes, drepanocytes, elliptocytes, leptocytes, schistocytes, spherocytes, and stomatocytes.

Red blood cells can also have abnormal inclusions, as a result of RNA deposits, precipitated nuclear material, or parasitic invasion. Special stains may be used to locate and define such inclusions. Such inclusions include basophilic stippling, Cabot rings, Heinz bodies, Howell-Jolly bodies, and Pappenheimer bodies. Red blood cells can also be invaded by parasites, especially a species of protozoans known as malarial parasites, called *Plasmodium* **species.**

Additional erythrocyte abnormalities include rouleau formation caused by an increase in plasma globulin, and red blood cell agglutination, which can be caused by incompatible blood being given during a transfusion and in patients with cold agglutinins.

Other testing in the hematology laboratory that directly concerns red blood cells includes hemoglobin testing. The hemoglobin level is a determination of the amount of oxygen-carrying capability of the red blood cells. The synthesis of hemoglobin requires the presence of iron, protoporphyrin IX, amino acids, RNA, and enzymes. Several methods have been used to determine the concentration of hemoglobin within blood. Today, hemoglobin results are automatically read on sophisticated cell counters.

The hematocrit (also referred to as Hct and packed cell volume) is a test to determine the ratio between the formed elements and the plasma after centrifugation. The erythrocyte sedimentation rate (ESR) is a test to determine the rate of fall of the red blood cells in a glass tube over a period of 1 hour. Red blood cell indices are calculations using the red blood cell count and hemoglobin and hematocrit values to help classify red cells as to size and hemoglobin count. Like the hematocrit, these indices are automatically calculated on automated cell counters.

REVIEW QUESTIONS

1. The immediate precursor cell of the metarubricyte (orthochromatic normoblast) is the
   a. reticulocyte
   b. rubricyte (polychromatic normoblast)
   c. prorubricyte (basophilic normoblast)
   d. erythrocyte

2. An erythrocytic cell with a pyknotic nucleus is the
   a. reticulocyte
   b. rubricyte (polychromatic normoblast)
   c. metarubricyte (orthochromatic normoblast)
   d. prorubricyte (basophilic normoblast)

3. An alteration in the shape of the erythrocyte is called
   a. anisocytosis
   b. poikilocytosis
   c. normocytosis
   d. normochromic

4. Red blood cells with blunt projections are
   a. burr cells
   b. blister cells
   c. dacryocytes
   d. drepanocytes

5. An individual who is homozygous for sickle cell anemia means
   a. the disease is not present
   b. the disease is present
   c. the disease will only show up with decreased oxygen pressure
   d. none of the above

6. Target cells are also called
   a. Mexican hat cells
   b. leptocytes
   c. codocytes
   d. all of the above

7. Completely round erythrocytes are
   a. incompatible with life
   b. never found in male patients
   c. an indication of spherocytic anemia
   d. never found in female patients

8. Which of the following are associated with the presence of RNA?
   a. reticulocytes
   b. basophilic stippling
   c. Pappenheimer bodies
   d. all of the above

9. Malaria is caused by
   a. bad luck
   b. a *Plasmodium* species
   c. an increase in hemoglobin
   d. a decrease in hemoglobin

10. Rouleau formation is caused by
    a drying the slides improperly
    b. an increase in Howell-Jolly bodies
    c. an increase in plasma globulin
    d. none of the above

11. To calculate the MCV, you would use the following formula
    a. hemoglobin (g/100 ml) × 10/red blood cell count
    b. standard deviation/mean × 100
    c. hemoglobin (g/100 ml)/hematocrit (%) × 10
    d. Hct (%) × 10/RBC (millions/cu mm)

12. The MCV is reported in
    a. g/dl
    b. fl
    c. pg
    d. percentage

13. The hematocrit represents the
    a. amount of red cells in one ml
    b. amount of hemoglobin in the RBC
    c. packed cell volume
    d. RBC divided by the Hb

14. The reticulocyte count is an expression of
    a. red cell width
    b. red cell hemoglobin concentration
    c. red cells in suspension
    d. red cell production

15. The normal value for a reticulocyte count is
    a. 0.5%–1.5%
    b. 3.0%–5.0%
    c. 0.1%–0.5%
    d. 10%–15%

16. The normal value for the MCH is
    a. 0.5%–1.5 %
    b. 80–100 fl
    c. 31–36 g/dl
    d. 27–31 pg
17. The typical erythrocyte measures _____ in diameter.
    a. 3 μ
    b. 3–5 μ
    c. 6.8–7.5 μ
    d. 8–10 μ
18. A hypochromic cell is seen as
    a. a red cell with complete dispersed hemoglobin
    b. a red cell with very little hemoglobin
    c. a red cell with only the middle showing hemoglobin
    d. a red cell with only the middle being empty
19. Anisocytosis is an indication of
    a. variation in shape
    b. variation in size
    c. variation in Hb concentration
    d. variation in nuclear mass

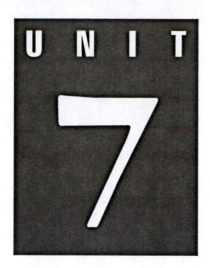

UNIT 7

Anemias and Hemoglobinopathies

Having completed this unit, it is the responsibility of the student to know the following:

- Define anemia.

- Identify anemia classifications.

- Stipulate which laboratory tests help identify the various anemias.

- Explain hemoglobinopathy.

- Stipulate which laboratory tests would help identify hemoglobinopathies.

GLOSSARY

gastrectomy removal of part or all of the stomach.

hemoglobinopathies inherited abnormalities in the structure of hemoglobin that result in hematological disorders.

homozygous possessing the same alleles for a given characteristic.

hypoxia reduction of oxygen supply to a tissue.

pancytopenia decrease in all cells produced in the bone marrow.

polychromatophilia affinity for a cell to accept many stains; red blood cells can stain many colors, especially when cells contain residual RNA.

polycythemia disorder due to increased production of red blood cells.

sprue chronic malabsorption syndrome.

INTRODUCTION

Anemia is defined as a reduced capacity to carry oxygen to the body tissues. The red blood cells (erythrocytes) have the important function of carrying oxygen to the tissues. Anemia can be caused by several factors. The red blood cells can be reduced due to a serious bleeding episode. Anemia can occur because the red cells are not being produced in normal quantities. It can also occur if the amount of hemoglobin produced is insufficient to fill the red cells. Anemia can result when the destruction of red cells exceeds production.

A healthy body can lose 20% of its blood volume without loss of body function (blood donations cause no problems for the healthy). If the blood loss is 30% to 40% of the total blood volume, then shock and circulatory collapse can be seen. If the loss reaches 50%, death can be imminent.

Anemia caused by loss of blood is first seen as "being tired." As the loss increases, muscle fatigue or weakness develops, possibly accompanied by a persistent headache. Fainting may also be common. With continued loss, the patient goes into coma because the brain is not receiving enough oxygen.

ANEMIA DIAGNOSIS

A laboratory test to determine the rate of red cell production is the *reticulocyte count*. This test can determine the effectiveness of production. It does not indicate the integrity of individual erythrocytes or how many are circulating in a given amount of blood. Tests that indicate the efficiency (ability to carry oxygen) of the red cells are the *hemoglobin test* as well as *red cell indices*. The red cell examination of the *differential* may be used to determine the variation in size and shape of the erythrocytes. The *red blood cell count* indicates the number of cells in circulation. Erythrocyte destruction can be tested by the *red cell fragility test* and also by the *bilirubin test* performed in the chemistry department of the clinical laboratory (the rest of the tests are performed in the hematology department).

All of these tests are useful in diagnosing anemia, with actual erythrocyte examination being one of the best indicators of anemia. Observing the smear will illustrate such phenomenon as hypochromia (decreased cellular hemoglobin), variations in size and shape (including diagnostic forms such as sickle cells), red cell inclusions, and **polychromatophilia** (red cells can appear bluish when not fully mature).

ANEMIA CLASSIFICATION

Anemias are classified in several ways. The cause of the anemia involved is called the *etiologic classification*. Variations in the size and shape of the erythrocytes are known as the *morphologic classification*.

ETIOLOGIC CLASSIFICATION

1. Anemias can be caused by an inherited gene, as seen in *thalassemia* and *hereditary spherocytosis*. A person with an inherited anemia will produce faulty red blood cells (along with some normal cells) that will not properly function.

2. Anemia can be caused by the inability of the bone marrow to produce enough cells that reach the peripheral circulation. This can take place because the bone marrow does not provide the raw materials for normal production as seen in *aplastic, iron-deficiency,* and *pernicious anemias.* These anemias can occur because of damage to the bone marrow, from lack of a proper diet, and so on.

3. Anemia can be caused by an increase in red cell destruction. If red blood cell membranes are faulty, the cells may rupture in the blood vessels just after entry. The cells may be attacked by the immune system, as in *hereditary spherocytic anemia, sickle cell, thalassemia major, erythroblastosis fetalis,* and *paroxysmal nocturnal hemoglobinuria.*

4. Anemia can be caused by a loss of red cells, as seen in the hemorrhagic anemias.

MORPHOLOGIC CLASSIFICATION

The morphologic classification is based on sizes and shapes of erythrocytes.

1. MACROCYTIC, NORMOCHROMIC red cells (larger than normal with normal color) are seen in *vitamin B$_{12}$* and *folic acid deficiency* and in *pernicious anemia.* These cells are also seen in liver disease, in **sprue,** and following a **gastrectomy.**

2. NORMOCYTIC, NORMOCHROMIC erythrocytes accompanying anemia can indicate retarded formation of red cells or the presence of tumor cells in the bone marrow. These cells are seen in *aplastic anemias,* the *leukemias, Hodgkin's disease, multiple myeloma,* metastatic cancers, and renal and inflammatory diseases. Normal appearing red blood cells also are present when cells have abnormal hemoglobins or increased destruction of red cells, as seen in *sickle cell anemia, paroxysmal nocturnal hemoglobinuria,* and *erythroblastosis fetalis.*

3. MICROCYTIC, HYPOCHROMIC erythrocytes are seen in *thalassemia, sideroblastic anemia,* and *iron-deficiency anemia.* Erythrocytes are smaller than normal and are often very pale, almost ghostly in appearance.

TYPES OF ANEMIA

Some of the more common anemias that may be seen in the clinical laboratory on a regular basis are listed below. For a more complete listing and discussion, a hematology reference textbook should be consulted.

IRON-DEFICIENCY ANEMIA

Iron-deficiency anemia is the most common anemia (Figure 7.1). It is most often caused by chronic or acute blood loss and is less commonly caused by insufficient intake of iron. The central portion of the hemoglobin molecule is iron (Figure 6.2), and the amount of hemoglobin available is dependent on the iron present. Sixty percent of the iron contained in the body is continually in circulation. Only pregnancy and childhood generally require an increased intake of iron. Males are able to withstand a decrease in intake longer than are females.

ANEMIA DUE TO BLOOD LOSS

Blood loss affects the red blood cell count and hemoglobin and hematocrit values, with severity depending on how much blood is lost. The reticulocyte population can take a few days to significantly increase in the peripheral circulation. A few nucleated red blood cells can be seen as well, depending again on how much blood has been lost. The white blood cell count is elevated almost immediately and can show a SHIFT TO THE LEFT. About 6 weeks after the episode, all values return to normal if the bleeding has stopped.

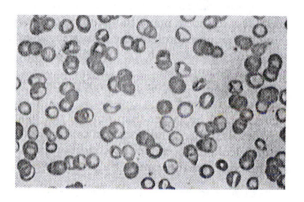

fig. 7.1. Iron-deficiency anemia. (From Marshall. *Fundamental Skills for the Clinical Laboratory Professional.* p. 337.)

E X E R C I S E **IRON-DEFICIENCY ANEMIA**

Purpose: To develop familiarity with red cell morphology consistent with iron-deficiency anemia.

Equipment Needed: Blood smears provided by the instructor

Procedure:
1. Bring the blood smear into focus using the oil immersion lens (100X).
2. Locate the thin portion of the smear where the red cells are just touching each other.
3. Make a drawing of several erythrocytes. Try to include all variations in the cells seen.

Besides the loss of cells, the initial decrease in levels of blood cells takes place also because of the body's attempt to make up for the loss of volume by an influx of tissue fluids. Increased reticulocyte counts indicate increased production, and white cell increases are because of reentry of white cells from the marginal pool. A shift to the left indicates increased production of white cells. The presence of polychromatophilia and nucleated erythrocytes indicates that the bone marrow is releasing immature red cells into circulation.

CHRONIC RENAL INSUFFICIENCY ANEMIA

This anemia is caused by kidney damage sufficient enough to reduce the production by the kidneys of the red blood cell stimulator *erythropoietin*. The red cells are usually normal looking, but the hematocrit is between 0.15 and 0.30 L/L. Burr cells may be seen in the smear because of a plasma factor that affects red cell metabolism, causing some hemolysis to occur. If the patient is in a dialysis program, macrocytes may be seen due to the loss of folic acid during dialysis. There are drugs on the market today that can stimulate the production of both red and white blood cells, with platelet stimulators ready to be marketed as well. These products have greatly improved the anemia status of dialysis patients.

ANEMIA OF CHRONIC DISORDERS

This type of anemia is found in chronic inflammations, infections, and neoplastic diseases. It is the second most common type of anemia. It is a difficult condition to diagnose because the reticulocyte count may be normal or slightly decreased. The hematocrit rarely is lower than 0.30 L/L, there is only a slight change in the size and shape of the red blood cells, and the serum iron level is only slightly decreased. The primary cause of the anemia must be treated to eliminate the anemic condition.

SIDEROBLASTIC ANEMIA

This anemia has two subtypes: *hereditary sideroblastic anemia* (a sex-linked recessive trait in males carried by females), and *acquired refractory sideroblastic anemia*.

In the hereditary form, a hematocrit of 0.20 L/L does not show up until puberty. The red cells show target cells and basophilic stippling, with slight anisocytosis and poikilocytosis. Erythrocytes are hypochromic and microcytic. The bone marrow illustrates many ringed sideroblasts, illustrating a defective heme production.

In the acquired form, the patients are usually over 50 with a hematocrit of 0.25 to 0.30 L/L. The red cells illustrate two populations: a large number of normocytic to macrocytic red cells and a smaller population of hypochromic red cells with heavy basophilic stippling. This form can develop as a response to a leukemia, alcoholism, lead poisoning, or tuberculosis therapy or can result in a myelodysplastic syndrome (refractory anemia with ringed sideroblasts).

APLASTIC ANEMIA

Aplastic anemia can occur as a congenital disease (called Fanconi's anemia), can be present because of damage to the bone marrow from physical or chemical agents, or the cause may not be known (idiopathic). Fanconi's anemia usually shows up between birth and age 8 years. Chemical causes include mustard compounds, benzene, arsenic, and drugs such as chloramphenicol, streptomycin, and sulfonamides. The laboratory shows a **pancytopenia**, with the differential showing anisocytosis and poikilocytosis. The reticulocyte count can be zero. There is usually a decrease in the white blood cells, but the smear can show a neutropenia and a lymphocytosis.

MEGALOBLASTIC ANEMIA

Megaloblastic anemias (also known as macrocytic anemias) are anemias that primarily are represented by anemia resulting from vitamin B_{12} or folic acid deficiency, or a combination of the two. There is abnormal red blood cell maturation in the bone marrow. Red blood cells can be larger with a more open chromatic pattern in the nucleus and often there is the presence of larger, hypersegmented neutrophils in the peripheral blood. The enlarged red blood cells (macrocytes) have MCV values of the order of 120 to 140 fl.

Pernicious anemia is most often found in persons over 60. The gastric mucosa cannot secrete *intrinsic factor* needed to aid in absorption of nutrients. This causes a vitamin B_{12} deficiency. Vitamin B_{12} is necessary for the normal production of red cells.

Antibodies can be found in this disorder that break down the intrinsic factor, pointing to an autoimmune component to this anemia. This would yield a marked anisocytosis and poikilocytosis. Basophilic stippling, Howell-Jolly bodies, and nucleated erythrocytes can also be seen in the smear. Neutrophils are hypersegmented and may be larger than normal.

One constant finding is a lack of free hydrochloric acid in the gastric secretions. There can be a slight increase in bilirubin. The iron level is normal.

EXERCISE **73** **PERNICIOUS ANEMIA**

Purpose: To recognize pernicious anemia in a differential smear.

Equipment Needed: Smears provided by the instructor.

Procedure:
1. Bring the blood smear into focus, using the low power initially, then using the oil immersion lens (100X).
2. Locate the thin portion of the smear where the red cells are just about touching.
3. Make a drawing of several erythrocytes seen. Include all variations in the cells seen.
4. How does this slide differ in appearance from a slide demonstrating iron-deficiency anemia?

Nutritional deficiencies can cause megaloblastic anemia. Deficiency of vitamin B_{12} is relatively rare in our society, but nutritional deficiency of folic acid can occur fairly commonly. It can be found in chronic alcoholism or in other conditions in which the diet is not well balanced. Folic acid 141deficiency is also observed when the requirement is increased in pregnancy, infancy, certain hemolytic anemias, and hyperthyroidism. The blood smears of these anemias resemble those of pernicious anemia.

THALASSEMIA

Thalassemia is a genetic disorder found in people native to the Mediterranean, Asian, and African areas. It is most often caused by the decreased production of the beta chains of the hemoglobin molecule (beta thalassemia). The chains that are produced are normal, but their numbers are reduced. In some cases, alpha chains are abnormal (alpha thalassemia). There are two forms of beta thalassemia: *thalassemia major* (Cooley's anemia) and *thalassemia minor* (Cooley's trait).

In beta thalassemia major, the individual is **homozygous** for the disease that appears in infancy. These individuals have a severe anemia. Their smear shows microcytic, hypochromic cells with marked anisocytosis and poikilocytosis. There is an increase in polychromatophilia, basophilic stippling, target cells, Howell-Jolly bodies, and siderocytes. The nucleated erythrocytes may be as high as 200 for every 100 WBC. There may be a slight shift to the left and a slight increase in the leukocyte count.

Beta thalassemia minor results from inheriting a single abnormal gene. This rarely results in a clinical disorder. The peripheral blood picture can show target cells and some poikilocytosis. Hemoglobin levels can be normal or slightly decreased. The MCH and MCV are slightly to moderately reduced. Serum iron levels may be slightly increased.

E X E R C I S E　 **74**　**IDENTIFICATION OF BETA THALASSEMIA MINOR**

SAFETY TECHNIQUE: WEAR GLOVES.

Purpose: The student observes the characteristic red blood cell picture on the differential smear of beta thalassemia minor.

Equipment: Blood smear provided by instructor.

Procedure:
1. Bring the blood smear into focus under low power first, then using the oil immersion lens (100X).
2. Locate the thin portion of the smear.
3. Notice the variety of shapes of red blood cells seen in the smear. Compare this picture with other anemia smears you have seen.
4. Draw all the variations that you see in this smear.

In beta thalassemia, the osmotic fragility test value is decreased. The rate of hemolysis is governed by the structure of the red cell. When the rate of hemolysis increases, the structure of the red cells is weaker, as seen in spherocytes. A decreased hemolysis is seen in cells where the amount of hemoglobin in the cells is small, as in thalassemia.

The osmotic fragility test is a measurement of cell shape and hemoglobin content, calculating how much water the cells can take in before they lyse. Spherocytes can take in little water, whereas hypochromic cells and targets cells can take in much more.

There are several quantitative tests that can be performed if the osmotic fragility screen in Exercise 75 is positive. Qualitative tests include the Sanford method, the Dacie method, the incubation method, and the Fragiligraph method. A reference textbook should be consulted to further study these methods.

HEREDITARY SPHEROCYTOSIS

This anemia is also known as congenital hemolytic anemia and is inherited as a non-sex linked dominant trait (rare cases can be recessive). The symptoms depend on the severity of the disease. As a general rule, the disease is more severe when it appears earlier in life. The red cells form spherocytes, the characteristic cell in the smear (Figure 6.6). Polychromatophilia with nucleated red blood cells and a reticulocyte count as high as 20% or more are a part of this anemia's blood picture. The osmotic fragility test is increased, and there are

---

E X E R C I S E   **75**   **OSMOTIC FRAGILITY TEST**

SAFETY TECHNIQUE: WEAR GLOVES.

Purpose: To become familiar with osmotic fragility testing. This is a screening test.

Equipment Needed: 0.5% and 0.85% sodium chloride solution, test tubes, distilled water, anticoagulated blood sample.

Procedure:
1. Set up four test tubes. Two are to be controls and two are to be tests.
2. Label tubes 0.5 NaCl test, 0.5 NaCl control, 0.85 test, 0.85 control.
3. Place 0.5 ml of blood to be tested in each.
4. Add 5 ml of respective solutions to each tube.
5. Invert to mix and centrifuge for 5 minutes.
6. If both patient tubes are clear and colorless, report the test as negative.
7. If the patient 0.5% tube shows a pink tinge, report the test as positive.

bilirubin and urobilinogen in the urine and stool. Removal of the spleen is a treatment for this anemia, since the spleen will destroy abnormal cells, rendering the patient seriously anemic.

HEMOLYTIC DISEASE OF THE NEWBORN (ERYTHROBLASTOSIS FETALIS)

Hemolytic disease of the newborn *(HDN)* is a disorder appearing in the infant at birth or soon after. Severe cases can affect the fetus before birth. HDN is caused by a blood incompatibility between the mother and infant. Whenever the infant's blood contains an antigen not found in the mother, the mother will develop antibodies against that antigen. In hemolytic disease of the newborn, the peripheral blood smear can show all stages of red cell maturation due to red blood cell destruction by the mother's antibodies. There is marked polychromatophilia, with the reticulocyte count being as high as 60%. There is an increase in leukocytes with immature forms seen in the differential. Bilirubin tests, indicative also of red blood cell destruction, may reach dangerously high levels.

Hemolytic disease of the newborn has been substantially reduced in the case of Rh incompatibility. A product called *Rh immune globulin* is given to Rh-negative mothers to prevent them from making antibodies to the Rh-negative fetus. A physician must order this product.

ABNORMAL HEMOGLOBIN

Hemoglobin transports respiratory gases, and the red blood cells transport hemoglobin. If there is an abnormal hemoglobin present, it is not capable of carrying oxygen as well as normal hemoglobin, which can result in a condition called **hypoxia.**

The structure of normal and abnormal hemoglobins after birth is based on four different types of polypeptide chains: alpha, beta, gamma, and delta. The production of these various chains is under genetic control. An abnormal hemoglobin may arise if only one amino acid substitution takes place.

THE STRUCTURE OF NORMAL HEMOGLOBIN

The major part of the normal hemoglobin is called Hb (hemoglobin) A. The globin part of the Hb A chains is composed of the two alpha chains, containing 141 amino acids each, and the two beta chains, containing 146 amino acids each. This Hb A is also designated $\alpha_2^A \beta_2^A$, meaning that there are two alpha chains and two beta chains in Hb A. This form of hemoglobin usually makes up 95% of the adult hemoglobin molecules.

A second type of normal hemoglobin found in the adult is Hb A_2, with a concentration of 1.5% to 3%. This hemoglobin type is also designated as $\alpha_2^A \delta_2^{A2}$. Ten amino acids differ in this hemoglobin.

Another type of normal hemoglobin in circulation is Hb F. This is the same fetal hemoglobin that supported life before birth and for about 1 to 2 years after birth. At birth, there is about 50% Hb F in circulation. It decreases until adulthood, when the level is less than 1%. This hemoglobin is designated as $\alpha_2^A \gamma_2^F$.

HEMOGLOBINOPATHIES

Inherited abnormalities in the amino acid sequence of the globin chains in hemoglobin that result in hematological disorders are known as **hemoglobinopathies.** These errors in hemoglobin structure can cause unstable hemoglobin that is unable to carry oxygen properly.

Hemoglobin S

Already discussed in Unit 6, this form of hemoglobin is a hereditary defect in the beta chain of hemoglobin that results in formation of intracellular crystals, distorting red blood cells into a sickled shape (see Figure 6.4). This sickling takes place under low oxygen conditions. This form of hemoglobin is designated as $\alpha_2{}^A \beta_2{}^{6valrs}$ (alpha two A, beta two, 6th position valine).

The disease does not show up in early life because of the predominance of Hb F. The sickled cells plug up small blood vessels and cause death to tissues because of lack of oxygen. The spleen atrophies in the adult. There is a decreased osmotic fragility test result. The red cell morphological examination usually shows target cells, Howell-Jolly bodies, nucleated RBCs, and of course sickled red cells. The heterozygous state is called the sickle cell trait. The red cells are only 20% to 40% Hb S. There may be no clinical signs, unless the individual is in an environment of reduced air pressure, such as flying in an unpressurized airplane. Target cells may be seen in the differential of sickle cell trait patients.

Sickle cell anemia is also evident using hemoglobin electrophoresis techniques.

Hemoglobin C

This type of hemoglobin is designated as $\alpha_2{}^A \beta_2{}^{6lys}$. It is found most often in African-Americans and is rarely seen in Caucasians. It can be inherited with hemoglobin S and has been found in both the homozygous and the heterozygous states (when inherited with hemoglobin S, an SC disease is produced, a double heterozygous state). In the red cell morphological examination, a high percentage of target cells is seen, sometimes as much as 90% of the cells. Hemoglobin C crystal forms have been seen in these cases if the cells are incubated with 3% (weight/volume) sodium chloride at body temperature (37°C) for 10 minutes. These crystals may also be seen in the Wright's stained smear after splenectomy. The crystal shape is like a small rod. The electrophoresis pattern indicates that almost 100% of the hemoglobin present is Hb C. Hemoglobin F may also be seen in the electrophoresis pattern, but usually less than 7% is present. These patients seem to live a normal life span.

Other Hemoglobin Forms

Hemoglobin D has several varieties that are indistinguishable from Hb S except by electrophoresis techniques. Abnormal alpha and beta chains have been detected. *Hemoglobin E* has the same electrophoretic pattern as hemoglobin A_2 and has been associated with a thalassemia with a blood picture slightly hypochromic and microcytic. Hemoglobin E is seen in the Southeast Asian population.

E X E R C I S E   76   SICKLEQUIK® TEST

SAFETY TECHNIQUE: WEAR GLOVES.

Purpose: To become familiar with the Diothionite method of sickle cell screening, using the Sicklequik® test.

Equipment Needed: Sicklequik® (General Diagnostics) kit; fresh whole blood or anticoagulated blood, test tube rack, centrifuge, control samples, latex gloves, biohazardous waste container.

Procedure:

1. Add 0.1 ml or 2 drops of whole blood to the Sicklequik reagent tube.
2. Recap tube and SHAKE VIGOROUSLY or vortex mix for 10 seconds.
3. Let stand in test tube rack for 5 minutes.
4. Centrifuge at 3400 rpm for 5 minutes.
5. If endpoint is not clear, recentrifuge.
6. Let stand vertically for 2 hours before reading results.
7. Several layers will form after centrifugation. Using the example below, read the tubes and controls. Follow kit directions carefully for reading results.
8. Dispose of all biohazardous wastes properly.

Hemoglobin H consists of four beta chains and no alpha chains. The deletion of three genes causes this defect. The individual shows a lifelong microcytic anemia, with the hemoglobin level between 8 and 10 g/dl and the MCV between 60 and 70 fl. There is a slightly elevated reticulocyte count, and the red cell morphological examination shows hypochromia, target cells, ovalocytes, and basophilic stippling. *Hemoglobin Bart's* is composed of four gamma chains that bind very quickly to oxygen. This feature does not allow this hemoglobin to be an oxygen transporter. Hemoglobin H and hemoglobin Bart's are seen in alpha thalassemias.

OTHER RED BLOOD CELL DISORDERS

POLYCYTHEMIA

Polycythemia is a disorder due to increased red blood cell production, analogous to leukemia in white blood cells. Also called erythremia, the cause of this disorder may be genetic, with some patients having hemoglobin variants. Some cases seem to have a neoplasm involving stem cell production.

There are two types of polycythemia, relative and absolute. Relative polycythemia is caused by a decrease in the plasma portion of the blood. The red blood cells are not actually increased, but the number of cells per unit volume is increased because of dehydration. Absolute polycythemia also has two subtypes: secondary and primary. The secondary type is caused by an increased level of erythropoietin in the blood attributed to any decrease in blood oxygen or to the presence of tumors. The primary type is also called *polycythemia vera* and is a chronic disease of persons over 60. It is characterized by an absolute increase in all cell lines, which increases the blood volume two to three times the normal volume. The plasma shows no change because of the increased cells; the patient therefore can have a purplish coloration to the skin. Increased platelets may cause coagulation problems. The peripheral blood smear shows polychromatophilia, with a few nucleated red blood cells and immature granulocytes present. Treatment includes therapeutic phlebotomies at regular intervals.

GLUCOSE-6-PHOSPHATE DEHYDROGENASE DEFICIENCY

Glucose-6-phosphate dehydrogenase deficiency *(G6PD)* is a sex-linked disease inherited on the X chromosome. G6PD is an enzyme present in red cells that plays a major role in the hexose monophosphate shunt. Complications can occur if compounds such as antimalarial drugs, sulfonamides, and analgesics are used. When these compounds are used, the absence of the G6PD enzyme can cause as many as 50% of the red blood cells to be destroyed.

PYRUVATE KINASE DEFICIENCY

Pyruvate kinase *(PK)* deficiency involves the deficiency of an enzyme involved in the glycolytic pathway. This inherited deficiency results in shortened red cell life spans. It is characterized by jaundice, splenomegaly, and anemia. The urine may be dark in color.

E X E R C I S E **POLYCYTHEMIA VERA**

Purpose: To observe a peripheral blood smear of a patient with polycythemia vera.

Equipment Needed: Smears provided by the instructor.

Procedure:
1. Bring the blood smear into focus, using the oil immersion lens (100X).
2. Locate the thin portion of the smear where the red cells are just touching each other.
3. Recognize as many immature red blood cell forms as you can see. Verify your identifications with the instructor.
4. Observe any red blood cell abnormalities that might be present.
5. Make a drawing of several erythrocytes.

SUMMARY

The decrease in the number of cells produced or in the ability of those cells to carry oxygen constitutes an anemia. Anemia can be caused by acute or chronic bleeding, by insufficient production of red blood cells for various reasons, by lack of hemoglobin to fill the cells, or by the destruction of red blood cells exceeding production.

The reticulocyte count can determine the effectiveness of new red blood cell production. It does not indicate the integrity of individual cells or how many are actually circulating. The hemoglobin test and the red blood cell indices are indicators of the efficiency of the red blood cells (ability to carry oxygen).

Anemias are classified by etiologic classification (cause) and by size and shape of the erythrocytes (morphologic). Anemias can be caused by an inherited gene (thalassemia), by the inability of the bone marrow to produce enough cells to reach the peripheral circulation (iron-deficiency anemia), by the increase in red cell destruction (sickle cell anemia), or by the loss of red blood cells (hemorrhagic anemias). Macrocytic, normochromic red cells are seen in vitamin B_{12} and folic acid deficiency. Normocytic, normochromic red blood cells accompanying anemia can indicate retarded red cell formation. Microcytic, hypochromic erythrocytes are seen in iron-deficiency anemia and thalassemia.

Specific types of anemia discussed in this unit include iron-deficiency anemia, blood loss anemia, chronic renal insufficiency anemia, sideroblastic anemia, aplastic anemia, megaloblastic anemia, thalassemia, hereditary spherocytosis, and hemolytic disease of the newborn.

Abnormal hemoglobin results in the red blood cell not carrying oxygen properly, which can result in hypoxia. Normal hemoglobin is called hemoglobin A, composed of two alpha chains and two beta chains. Adults also have hemoglobin A_2, found in small amounts. Hemoglobin F supports life before birth and for about 1 to 2 years after birth. In the adult, it makes up less than 1% of hemoglobin.

Hemoglobinopathies are inherited abnormalities in amino acid sequences that result in hematological disorders. Some of these disorders include hemoglobin S (causing sickle cell anemia), hemoglobin C, and other forms. Other red blood cell disorders include polycythemia, glucose-6-phosphate dehydrogenase deficiency (G6PD), and pyruvate kinase deficiency.

REVIEW QUESTIONS

1. What is polychromatophilia?
   a. a form of hereditary anemia
   b. a condition caused by a decreased production of membrane proteins
   c. a bluish coloration of RBCs due to residual RNA
   d. an observable decrease in RBC hemoglobin content
2. Of the following, which would be difficult to detect if only the red cell morphology was used?
   a. macrocytic, normochromic anemia
   b. normocytic, normochromic anemia
   c. microcytic, hypochromic anemia
   d. microcytic, hyperchromia anemia
3. Which of the following could show up in children due to lead poisoning?
   a. aplastic anemia
   b. anemia of chronic disorders
   c. hereditary sideroblastic anemia
   d. acquired sideroblastic anemia
4. Hemolytic disease of the newborn is caused by
   a. a genetic defect
   b. an blood incompatibility
   c. an acute aplastic anemia
   d. a renal disorder
5. Polycythemia vera is characterized by
   a. a pancytopenia
   b. absolute increases in all cell lines
   c. absolute increases in one cell line
   d. none of the above
6. Of the following, which has red cell shape that changes if there is a decrease in oxygen pressure?
   a. sickle cell anemia
   b. thalassemia major
   c. thalassemia minor
   d. polycythemia vera
7. Of the following, which is found in normal adult blood?
   a. Hb A
   b. Hb A_2
   c. Hb F
   d. all of the above
8. What deficiencies are associated with megaloblastic anemias?
   a. iron
   b. vitamin A
   c. vitamin B_{12} and folic acid
   d. vitamin C

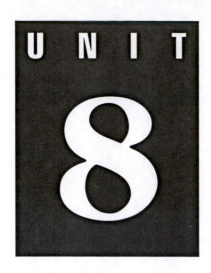

UNIT 8

Hemostasis and Coagulation Procedures

LEARNING OBJECTIVES

Having completed this unit, it is the responsibility of the student to know the following:

- Identify the two types of hemostasis.

- Describe the structure of the platelet and its changes during primary hemostasis.

- Identify laboratory tests associated with primary hemostasis, being aware of normal test values.

- Identify the two pathways associated with secondary hemostasis and describe the circumstances under which each pathway is employed.

- Describe the activity of the factors associated with secondary hemostasis.

- Discuss the significance of fibrinolysis.

- Identify some causes of circulating anticoagulants and hypercoagulable states.

- Identify laboratory tests associated with secondary hemostasis, being aware of normal test values.

GLOSSARY

activated partial thromboplastin time abbreviated APTT; common coagulation test to assess the intrinsic coagulation mechanism.

activation referring to platelets, the process by which platelets change shape and attract other platelets to do the same.

adhesion process in which platelets attach to the collagen fibers (a form of connective tissue).

coagulation factors blood clotting factors that are present in the body in an inactive form until stimulated to aid in coagulation.

DIC disseminated intravascular coagulation; condition accompanied by sudden, dramatic stimulus of coagulation throughout the body.

extrinsic pathway one of two pathways (intrinsic pathway being the other) involved in blood coagulation leading to fibrin formation; includes factors VII, X, V, II, and I.

fibrin insoluble protein essential to blood clotting.

fibrinogen soluble precursor of the clot-forming protein fibrin; plasma protein manufactured by the liver.

fibrinolysis process by which the clot is dissolved after bleeding has stopped.

hemostasis cessation of bleeding.

hypercoagulability abnormally increased coagulation of the blood.

intrinsic pathway one of two pathways (extrinsic pathway being the other) involved in blood coagulation leading to fibrin formation; includes factors XII, Fletcher, Fitzgerald, XI, IX, VIII, X, V, II, and I.

megakaryocyte largest cell found within the bone marrow that produces platelets.

petechiae small purplish-red spot appearing under skin due to hemorrhage; indicative of platelet reduction or malfunction.

platelet portion of a megakaryocyte that adheres to foreign surfaces to form aggregates in response to tissue and blood vessel injuries.

platelet aggregation process by which platelets stick together in a mass to form a platelet plug.

prothrombin time abbreviated PT; common coagulation test to assess the extrinsic coagulation system; commonly used to monitor oral anticoagulant therapy.

thrombocyte technical name for a platelet.

thrombosis clot formation within a blood vessel.

INTRODUCTION

Obtaining a blood sample from a patient produces a puncture wound. The flow of blood must be halted. After the specimen is obtained, a sterile gauze pad is placed over the wound with pressure applied by either the patient or blood drawer. Sometimes patients are asked to raise their arm towards the head while applying pressure. This unit deals with the series of reactions that take place to halt the flow of blood.

Two aspects of the complicated process of coagulation are recognized. *Primary hemostasis* involves the initial changes and responses when an insult to blood vessels occurs. Blood vessels will constrict immediately when damaged. **Platelets** secrete chemicals as they stick to the margins in the wall of the injured vessel.

Secondary hemostasis involves a complex sequence of physiochemical reactions in the body. The plug of the bleeding is initiated by the primary system but is reinforced by the secondary system. Each system will be considered separately. Testing takes place for each system as well.

The diagnostic technology available in hemostasis has grown rapidly. The emphasis today on preventative medicine has led the medical profession to look for genetic and acquired problems with coagulation (coagulopathies) early in one's life so that bleeding problems and resultant medical costs can be curbed in later years. Rapid turnaround time using modern automated instruments makes coagulation testing an important part of trauma medicine.

PRIMARY HEMOSTASIS

Any damage to a vein brings on a constriction in the smooth (visceral) muscle fibers associated with the veins' structure. This reduces the flow of blood to minimize blood loss. This first step is the beginning of a process called primary hemostasis.

To understand the next step in **hemostasis**, the student should be aware of the anatomy and physiology of the **thrombocyte** (platelet). Technically the platelet is not a cell, but is bit of cytoplasm of a **megakaryocyte**. A platelet is about 2 to 4 μ in diameter. The megakaryocyte normally is retained in the bone marrow and is not normally found in the peripheral circulation. If, however, it is found in the bloodstream, a bone may have been broken, as in a compound fracture, and the marrow could have escaped its normal confines.

Platelet morphology is illustrated in Figure 8.1. A platelet resembles a disc that has many small holes and channels extending deeply into the interior. The platelet is divided into four parts, each with its own particular anatomy and function. The *peripheral layer* consists of an outer membrane surrounded by glycoproteins, called the *glycocalyx* (biphospholipid layer with embedded proteins). Some glycoproteins cause platelet activation. *Arachidonic acid* is a major part of the membrane and causes vasoconstriction and platelet aggregation.

The *microtubule layer* (the sol gel zone) consists of microscopic tubes used to maintain the disc shape of the platelet. This layer also includes contracting proteins called *actin* and *myosin*. They can change the shape of the platelet. The microtubule layer forms the cytoskeleton of the platelet.

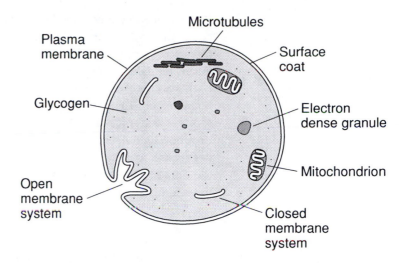

fig. 8.1. Platelet morphology. (From Marshall. *Fundamental Skills for the Clinical Laboratory Professional.* p. 429.)

The *organelle layer* is beneath the microtubule layer. It consists of *mitochondria* (producers of ATP, a source of cellular energy), *glycogen* (breaking down glucose to release energy), *lysosomes* (containing hydrolytic enzymes), *alpha granules* (containing two groups of proteins), and *dense bodies* (consisting of ATP, ADP, phosphate compounds, calcium ions, and serotonin—a vasoconstrictor).

The *membrane systems* are the innermost layer, consisting of passageways from the surface to the interior. Here calcium ions are stored that are needed for platelet metabolism and activation.

THE PLATELET PLUG

One of the major roles of the platelet is to form a plug when small holes appear in blood vessels. Platelets attach to the exposed collagen fibers (a form of connective tissue) in a process called **adhesion**. They begin to change shape, using the microfilaments and the energy source ATP. This process is called **activation**. When the platelet changes shape, it attracts other platelets to change shape and stick together (called **platelet aggregation**) that produces a platelet plug. Once activated, this is a continuous process, but it can be reversed if the stimulus is not strong enough.

PLATELET ASSESSMENT

The platelet count is of vital importance when the physician is assessing a patient's coagulation system. If a decrease in platelets is found, the patient is at risk for uncontrolled bleeding.

Platelets are difficult to count because of their small size. They can often be mistaken for artifacts. There are several methods employed in determining the platelet count. Indirect methods include the Fonio method and the platelet estimation. These indirect methods are estimates and should not be used if direct methods are available.

The most common method today of platelet determination is by automated cell counters (see Unit 9). Platelet counts are included as a part of an entire battery of cell counting. Other less automated direct methods include the Rees and Ecker, the Brecher-Cronkite, and the Unopette method (Exercise 78).

Direct methods require the dilution of a blood sample. The direct platelet count is performed manually by using a light microscope (a phase contrast microscope is better for visualizing the platelets). To perform a direct method using the common light microscope, the light passing through the microscope condenser is decreased, making it possible to see the tiny platelets. It is also necessary to allow the diluted blood to stand for a short period of time for the platelets to settle in the counting chamber.

EXERCISE 78 UNOPETTE® SYSTEM FOR PLATELET COUNTING

SAFETY TECHNIQUE: WEAR GLOVES. PERFORM A FINGER PUNCTURE SAFELY, ALWAYS FOLLOWING BLOOD HANDLING PRECAUTIONS.

Purpose: The Unopette® system utilizes a 1% ammonium oxalate solution that hemolyses red cells. The platelets are counted using a counting chamber and microscope.

Equipment Needed: Unopette® system, counting chamber, microscope, fingerstick equipment, biohazard disposal container.

Procedure:
1. Obtain a Unopette® system, consisting of the reservoir with premeasured diluent, a cap shield used to puncture the reservoir, and a capillary tube of uniform bore size (Figure 4.5).
2. Following the directions that accompany the Unopette® system, perform a finger puncture on a fellow student. Be sure to follow appropriate procedures under the supervision of your instructor.
3. Puncture the reservoir with the shield.
4. Touch the capillary tube to the flow of blood from the finger punctured until the tube fills. It will not overfill.
5. Squeeze the Unopette® reservoir. After wiping the outside of the capillary tube of excess blood, insert the tube into the diluent solution. Release the pressure on the sides of the reservoir, drawing in the blood. Rinse several times. ALWAYS FOLLOW PRECAUTIONS RELATING TO SAFE HANDLING OF BLOOD PRODUCTS!
6. Reverse the position of the capillary tube and attach it to the reservoir. Mix the contents by rolling the reservoir between gloved hands for several seconds.

E X E R C I S E   **78** UNOPETTE® SYSTEM FOR PLATELET
COUNTING *(continued)*

7. Allow 10 minutes for complete hemolysis of the red blood cells to occur.
8. Charge a hemocytometer and allow 5 minutes for settling.
9. Count the center area and the four corners of the central area (RBC area) of the chamber.
10. Carefully dispose of all biohazardous waste.
11. Calculate the number of platelets by:
    Number of platelets counted × the dilution correction (100) × volume correction (10) divided by 1.
    NORMAL VALUES: 150 to 400 × 10^9/L

A decrease in the number of platelets can result in blood entering the tissues. This blood forms small purple spots called **petechiae** (caused by high venous blood pressure) or larger bruises (3 mm or larger) called *ecchymoses*. The capillary fragility test measures the ability of capillaries to withstand increased stress, reflecting the integrity of vessel walls and the maintenance activities of platelets.

E X E R C I S E **79** CAPILLARY FRAGILITY TEST

SAFETY TECHNIQUE: WEAR GLOVES.

Purpose: This test, also called the Rumpel-Leede test or the tourniquet test, tests the ability of the capillaries to resist pressure not more than 100 mm Hg.

Equipment Needed: A marking pen and a blood pressure apparatus.

Procedure:
1. Take the marking pen and mark any tiny hemorrhages already present before the test. Disregard these spots.
2. Just above the elbow, wrap the blood pressure apparatus and inflate to halfway between the systolic and diastolic pressure, but not more than 100 mm Hg (your instructor may want to give a demonstration of the use of the blood pressure apparatus before proceeding).
3. Three inches below the blood pressure apparatus, draw a circle about 1.5 inches in diameter to establish the test area.
4. Maintain pressure for 5 minutes.

EXERCISE   **79**   CAPILLARY FRAGILITY TEST *(continued)*

5. Release the pressure cuff and allow 15 minutes to elapse.
6. Observe for any petechiae on the arm. Disregard any found within ½ inch of the blood pressure cuff.
7. If less than ten fresh petechiae are found, report the test as NEGATIVE.
8. If ten to twenty fresh petechiae are found, report the test as BORDERLINE.
9. If more than twenty fresh petechiae are found, report the test as POSITIVE.

Some Conditions Associated with a Positive Capillary Resistance Test

Purpura hemorrhagica	Aplastic anemia
Chronic nephritis	Scurvy
Purpura simplex	Measles
Hypofibrinogenemia	Scarlet fever
Vitamin K deficiency	Achylia gastrica

BLEEDING TIME TESTING

There are a number of different test that have been used to test for primary hemostasis. Bleeding time testing is helpful to detect vascular abnormalities and platelet abnormalities or deficiencies.

Two methods are commonly used for bleeding time testing: the Duke method and the Ivy method. The Duke method is less popular and involves puncturing the rounded, fatty portion of the earlobe. The Ivy method, which is similar to the Duke method, is described in Exercise 80. Bleeding tests should be performed only after the patient has abstained from taking aspirin for 3 days.

The standardized Simplate® method is the method of choice when performing the Ivy method. It uses a cutting device (Figure 8.2) that is spring loaded with one or two blades.

Some Conditions Associated with a Prolonged Bleeding Time Test

Very low platelet levels

Aspirin ingestion within the past few days

Platelet dysfunction syndromes

von Willebrand's disease and severe fibrinogen deficiency

Abnormalities in walls of small blood vessels

Disseminated intravascular coagulation (DIC)

Severe liver disease

Leukemias

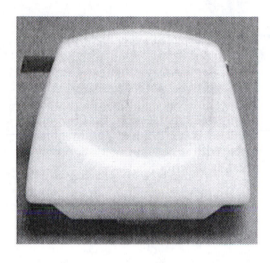

fig. 8.2. Ivy bleeding template. (From Marshall. *Fundamental Skills for the Clinical Laboratory Professional.* p. 454.)

E X E R C I S E **80** **IVY BLEEDING TIME TEST (SIMPLATE® METHOD)**

SAFETY TECHNIQUE: WEAR GLOVES. TAKE SPECIAL PRECAUTIONS WHEN USING DEVICES WITH BLADES.

Purpose: A constant pressure is applied above the elbow by using a blood pressure cuff. The volar surface of the forearm is cut, with bleeding timed until cessation.

Equipment Needed: Stopwatch, Simplate® bleeding time device (other brands such as Surgicutt® can also be used), blood pressure cuff, sterile gauze or filter paper, butterfly bandage, alcohol swabs, biohazard waste container.

Procedure:
1. Select a site on the volar surface (palm side) of the patient's arm, cleansing it with an alcohol swab.
2. Place the blood pressure cuff above the elbow and inflate it to 40 mm Hg (20 mm Hg for newborns) while the volar surface is air drying.
3. Break off the safety device on the bleeding time blade unit and place it in the clean area within 30 seconds after inflating the blood pressure cuff. Be sure to use precautions when dealing with a bladed instrument.
4. When ready, push the trigger to release the blade(s) and start the stopwatch.

E X E R C I S E **80** **IVY BLEEDING TIME TEST (SIMPLATE® METHOD)** *(continued)*

5. Without using any pressure, bring the filter paper/gauze to the puncture every 30 seconds until no fresh blood appears.
6. Turn off the stopwatch.
7. Place a butterfly bandage over the wound and advise the patient to keep the bandage on for 24 hours.
8. Dispose of all biohazardous wastes properly.
9. Report the results as:
   Bleeding time = _____ minutes _____ seconds
   (Simplate® and Surgicutt® methods normal results 2 to 9.5 minutes)

Note: This test can leave scars if cuts are made across the lines of tension. The cutting device should be placed in a horizontal fashion on the volar surface of the forearm. With proper bandaging, only a slight scar should result.

CLOT RETRACTION TESTING

When placed in a test tube, whole blood will clot and begin to retract from the sides of the test tube, observable after 1 hour and 50% complete in 4 hours. This is a test to determine the functioning of the platelets as well as an indication of their quantity.

E X E R C I S E **81** **CLOT RETRACTION TEST**

SAFETY TECHNIQUE: WEAR GLOVES. USE PROPER PRECAUTIONS WHEN PERFORMING A VENIPUNCTURE.

Purpose: Normal blood will clot completely, with retraction of the clot beginning in 1 hour. By the end of 24 hours, a normal clot should have retracted completely. Incomplete retraction suggests a low platelet count or poorly functioning platelets.

Equipment Needed: Phlebotomy equipment, silicone-coated test tube, 37°C incubator, timer, biohazard container.

Procedure:
1. Perform a venipuncture using a silicone-coated tube.
2. Not disturbing the tube, place it in a 37°C incubator, observing after 1 hour.

E X E R C I S E   81   CLOT RETRACTION TEST *(continued)*

3. Note if the clot is retracted from the sides of the tube, the bottom only, or both.
4. Replace in incubator and check at 2 and 4 hours.
5. Recheck in 24 hours.
   Report as: NORMAL RETRACTION if in 2 to 4 hours it is nearly complete and if in 24 hours it is completely retracted from the bottom and sides of the tube.

Note: This test IS NOT a sensitive measure of platelet dysfunction.

Some Conditions that can Show an Abnormality in the Clot Retraction Time

Thrombocytopenia	Aplastic anemia
Purpura hemorrhagica	Acute leukemia
Glanzmann's disease	Multiple myeloma
Hodgkin's disease	Polycythemia

PLATELET AGGREGATION STUDIES

This testing is not a routine platelet screening test. Platelet aggregation studies are performed to detect abnormalities in platelet aggregation. Platelet aggregation is reduced in infectious mononucleosis, acute leukemia, aspirin use, von Willebrand's disease, and other disorders. This testing is thoroughly explained in hematology reference textbooks.

SECONDARY HEMOSTASIS

The ability to stop the flow of blood in a more stabilized fashion is the realm of secondary hemostasis. This process is also known as the fibrin-forming system. This system is mediated by many coagulation proteins normally present in the blood in an inactive state (Table 8.1). The term secondary hemostasis is used to define the coagulation factor's role in the hemostatic mechanism. All coagulation proteins are produced in the liver, with the possible exception of factor VIII. When the liver is severely diseased (alcoholism can destroy the liver), coagulation problems will almost always occur. Almost all factors have been given a Roman numeral to designate their discovery sequence in the coagulation process. Many have retained their original names because of common usage.

The **coagulation factors** first act as substrates. When activated, they act as enzymes to carry on the reaction. Each coagulation factor has its particular function in the overall reactions. If a factor is missing or not functioning properly, the clot will not form properly, as seen in hemophilia. Most factors are produced in the liver.

Table 8.1. Coagulation Factors

Factor	Name	Synonym
I	Fibrinogen	
II	Prothrombin	
III	Thromboplastin	
IV	Calcium	
V	Proaccelerin	Labile factor
VII	Proconvertin	Stable factor
VIII	Antihemophilic factor	Antihemophilic globulin, antihemophilic factor A
IX	Plasma thromboplastin component	Christmas factor, antihemophilic factor B
X	Stuart factor	Prower factor
XI	Plasma thromboplastin antecedent	Antihemophilic factor C
XII	Hageman factor	Glass or contact factor
XIII	Fibrinase	Fibrin-stablilizing factor
	Fitzgerald factor	High molecular weight kininogen (HMWK)
	Fletcher factor	Prekallikrein

The sequences of activity in secondary hemostasis involve two interrelated systems. The first is called the **extrinsic pathway**. The extrinsic pathway includes interactions of factors I, II, V, VII, and X reacting to cause a chemical conversion that aids the clotting mechanism.

The intrinsic system is sometimes activated merely by platelets coming in contact with a rough surface. This system involves factors I, II, V, VIII, IX, X, XI, XII, the Fitzgerald factor, and the Fletcher factor interacting together to also aid clotting. The interaction of these systems to aid the coagulation process is called the *Waterfall Theory of Coagulation.* Figure 8.3 illustrates this theory. A better understanding of these complex phenomena can be found in hematology reference textbooks.

FACTOR SCREENING TESTS

A variety of manual, semiautomated, and automated techniques are used to assess quantity and quality of clotting factors in the blood. The standard anticoagulant used for screening tests and factor assays is 3.8% trisodium citrate, a blue-topped tube.

Blood taken for coagulation studies must be collected with particular care to avoid trauma so that substances involved in blood coagulation are not altered. Blood should be drawn with a clean, carefully executed venipuncture. Hemolyzed blood can result in unreliable and misleading coagulation results. The collection tube also must be *completely filled* to maintain the correct ratio of anticoagulant to blood. If multiple vials are drawn, samples for coagulation studies should be drawn last. When a person with bleeding tendencies is being tested, care should be taken to apply pressure on the venipuncture site continuously until bleeding has stopped.

LEE AND WHITE WHOLE BLOOD CLOTTING TIME

Historically, a simple method of determining blood clotting has been the Lee and White whole blood clotting time. This test is prolonged, with severe defects in the

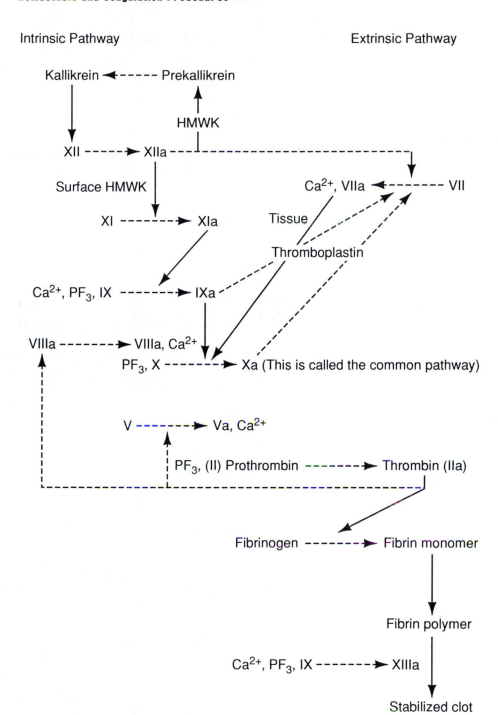

fig. 8.3. Waterfall theory of coagulation.

intrinsic and extrinsic coagulation systems and with anticoagulants circulating in the blood. Traditionally, this test was used as a monitor for anticoagulant drug therapy. However, today the test is found to be more inaccurate than modern tests, and blood exposure for the technician is excessive. It is no longer used in most facilities.

THE PROTHROMBIN TIME

The most frequently ordered coagulation test, the **prothrombin time (PT)** is the time required to form a fibrin clot when plasma is added to a thromboplastin-calcium mixture. This test measures the extrinsic pathway of coagulation involving factors II, V, VII, and X, as well as fibrinogen. This test is also extremely helpful in monitoring oral anticoagulant therapy. Patients often have prothrombin times measured weekly to monitor their medication.

The prothrombin time is performed on automated coagulation instruments in many laboratories today. Exercise 82 illustrates a fibrometer method of performing this testing, used by some facilities as a backup method to more automated instruments. This instrument, as well as more automated coagulation instrumentation, is discussed in Unit 9.

E X E R C I S E      ## THE PROTHROMBIN TIME (FIBROMETER METHOD)

SAFETY TECHNIQUE: WEAR GLOVES.

Purpose: The fibrometer is an instrument that measures electrical impedance by formation of a fibrin clot.

Equipment Needed: Fibrometer, sodium citrate blood samples (blue-stoppered blood tube), normal and abnormal control plasma, coagulation reagents, pipette tips, soft laboratory tissues, specimen cups, biohazard disposal container.

Procedure:

1. Place several sample cups in the thermal prep block (heating block) to warm. Turn the instrument on.
2. Using the attached pipettor, turn the plunger volume adjustor and set it to 0.2 ml.
3. Using a disposable plastic pipette tip, pipette exactly 0.2 ml of reagent into the sample cups to warm for at least 5 minutes. Clean off any excess from outside of pipette using soft laboratory tissue.
4. Place a sample cup in the reactor well.
5. Push the digital readout reset button so that all digits read zero.
6. Turn the plunger volume adjustor and set it to 0.1 ml. Use a clean pipette tip for each sample.
7. Draw up 0.1 ml volume of normal control plasma.
8. Make sure to wipe off excess plasma from outside of the tip.
9. Adjust the probe arm so that it is directly over the specimen cup in the reactor well.
10. Place the pipette tip at the top of the sample cup and push the plunger completely in. The probe arm will drop into the cup and the timer will start.

EXERCISE ▮82▮ THE PROTHROMBIN TIME (FIBROMETER METHOD) (continued)

11. When the probe is stopped from moving by the formation of a fibrin clot, the timer will stop.
12. Record the results and repeat the test. Make sure that your results are within acceptable ranges of each other. You have run prothrombin time testing on the control.
13. Perform similar techniques using the abnormal control and the patient plasma. Record your results. Prothrombin time = _____ seconds.
14. Dispose of all biohazardous wastes properly.

Note: Normal prothrombin time is 12 to 14 seconds. Each laboratory develops its own "normal" range. The preferred method of reporting the patient's prothrombin result is to report the result in seconds and comparing that time with the normal control time, also reported in seconds. This test is prolonged in individuals with a factor deficiency or deficiencies. It is also prolonged in the presence of circulating anticoagulants such as FDPs and heparin.

Some problems that can be encountered when performing the prothrombin time are listed below.

- The test is not performed within an hour after collection.
- The sample can be contaminated with tissue thromboplastin when a venipuncture is not clean.
- If a syringe is used for the venipuncture, air bubbles could mix with the blood, resulting in inaccurate results.
- The plasma may not be spun down and separated properly from the red blood cells.
- The sodium citrate tube may not be filled completely, causing an improper dilution of blood with the anticoagulant.

Some Conditions that can Show an Increase in the Prothrombin Time

Vitamin K deficiency	Anticoagulant therapy
Specific factor deficiencies	Certain liver diseases
Disseminated intravascular coagulation (DIC)	Presence of fibrin split products (FSP)

THE ACTIVATED PARTIAL THROMBOPLASTIN TIME (APTT)

This test is used to detect disorders in the intrinsic clotting system. It can also be used to detect the presence of circulating coagulation inhibitors (circulating anticoagulants) and for monitoring anticoagulant therapy using heparin.

Table 8.2. Normal Values for Selected Coagulation Tests

Test	Normal Value
Platelet count	150,000–450,000/mm³
Ivy bleeding time (Simplate®)	2.3–9.5 minutes
Clot retraction	50%–100% 2 hours
Platelet aggregation	Full response to ADP, epinephrine, and collagen
Prothrombin time (PT)	Less than 2-second deviation from control: 12–14 seconds
Activated partial thromboplastin time (APTT)	< 35 seconds
Fibrinogen assay	200–400 mg/dl
Factor assays	Factor VII: 65%–135% of normal Factor VIII: 70%–150% Factor IX: 60%–140% Factor X: 45%–155% Factor XI: 65%–135% Factor XII: 50%–150%
D-Dimer	<0.5 µg/ml
Fibrin(ogen) products	Degradation 4.9± 2.8 µg FDP/ml
Thrombin time	15 seconds

The performance of this test requires using a partial thromboplastin reagent to which an activator has been added as well as a calcium chloride solution to ensure the presence of calcium ions in the coagulation process. This test is also performed in most laboratories by automated equipment.

If both the PT and the APTT are prolonged, the coagulation problem could be in a common pathway in the intrinsic and extrinsic system. If the APTT is prolonged and the PT is normal, the problem could be in the intrinsic pathway. If the APTT is normal and the PT is prolonged, the problem is usually with factor VII in the extrinsic pathway.

FACTOR ASSAYS

Factor assays are performed in the investigation of inherited and acquired bleeding disorders. When either the prothrombin time and the activated partial thromboplastin time are both prolonged or one is prolonged, the physician may ask the clinical laboratory to further test the patient to determine the factor involved in the bleeding problem. These tests are described in detail in hematology reference textbooks.

Hemophilia

Hemophilia refers to specific hereditary disorders caused by deficiencies of clotting factors. The most common hemophilia is factor VIII deficiency, known as hemophilia A. This disorder occurs in one per 10,000 live male births. Hemophilia A is a sex-linked disorder. Patients have spontaneous bleeding episodes, with some developing chronic complications such as bleeding and arthritis. Patients receive concentrated, freeze-dried factor VIII to stop bleeding. Figure 8.4 traces the inheritance of hemophilia.

Other factor testing encountered in the clinical laboratory can include testing for von Willebrand's disease that involves factor VIII as well, and factor IX deficiency, also called hemophilia B or Christmas factor. Students are encouraged to read further about factor deficiencies.

EXERCISE OBSERVATION OF AUTOMATED COAGULATION TESTING

Purpose: The student observes automated coagulation equipment in a clinical laboratory setting to gain insight into coagulation testing.

Procedure:

1. If feasible, your instructor will arrange a field trip to a local clinical laboratory for student observation of automated coagulation equipment (you may be assigned to arrange a visitation of a coagulation laboratory on your own).

2. During your visit, ask if you may observe testing for the prothrombin time (PT) and the **activated partial thromboplastin time (APTT).**

3. Find out what the backup methods are for these two common tests if the instrument used to perform these tests is not functioning.

4. Find out what other coagulation tests are *routinely* run in the department. If time permits, observe other routine testing.

5. Inquire about less routinely run tests. How are factor tests performed?

6. What coagulation testing is sent to another laboratory for testing?

7. If possible, obtain a fee schedule for coagulation testing.

8. Is there a reference laboratory in your area that specializes in coagulation testing? Find out what tests are performed in that laboratory.

THROMBIN TIME

The *thrombin time* is a test used to detect a condition known as hypofibrinogenemia (little fibrinogen is present in the plasma) and dysfibrinogenemia (abnormal fibrinogen molecule). This test is also abnormal if a patient is on heparin therapy. Thrombin times can also be performed on automated equipment.

FIBRINOGEN ASSAY

The *fibrinogen assay* is used to detect afibrinogenemia and hypofibrinogenemia, two diseases that are characterized by decreased fibrinogen levels. Another disease state called dysfibrinogenemia may have normal amounts of fibrinogen, but it does not function normally. Fibrin clots will be decreased.

FIBRINOLYSIS

Besides having a system for clot formation, the body also has a means by which the clot may be removed. This mechanism is not fully understood.

As soon as clotting has begun, **fibrinolysis** is initiated to break down the clot that has formed. Normally, this system functions to keep the vascular system free

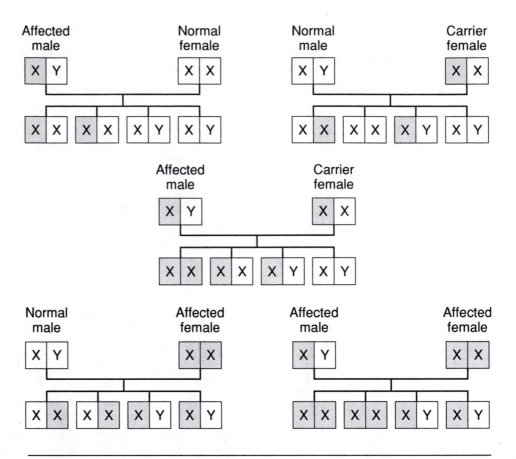

fig. 8.4. Inheritance of hemophilia. (From Marshall. *Fundamental Skills for the Clinical Laboratory Professional.* p. 436.)

EXERCISE 84 HEMOPHILIA A

Purpose: The student researches hemophilia A to understand the seriousness of an inherited coagulation disorder.

Procedure:

The student answers the following questions:

1. Briefly describe hemophilia A. Who gets this disease? How does it differ from von Willebrand's disease? Review Figure 8.4.
2. What tests are run in the clinical laboratory to diagnose this disorder?
3. What product does the hemophiliac receive from the blood bank in the clinical laboratory?
4. Why have so many hemophiliacs contracted AIDS in the 1980s?
5. Name and briefly describe hemophilia B.

of fibrin clots or deposited fibrin. The fibrinolytic system and the coagulation system are in equilibrium in the normal person.

There are many tests to assess the functioning of this important system, including:

- *Fibrin-degradation products* When human fibrin is digested, several large and small degradation products result. These products are broken down by the liver and excreted by the kidneys. If such products are present in increasing amounts, it is assumed that a clotting process is taking place.
- *D-Dimer* This test is a simple latex agglutination test to detect D-dimer, signifying the presence of plasmin plus thrombin. It takes plasmin to create the D fragment, and thrombin is required to activate factor XIII to factor XIIIa to cross-link the D fragments. This test is replacing fibrinogen and fibrin degradation products to help diagnose disseminated intravascular coagulation, discussed in the next section.

DISSEMINATED INTRAVASCULAR COAGULATION

Disseminated intravascular coagulation (DIC) is a serious condition in which hemostasis mechanisms are activated, causing intravascular fibrin production and consequent fibrinolysis. DIC accompanies various clinical conditions, including:

- *Obstetrical problems,* including amniotic fluid clots, abruptio placentae, toxemia, and retained dead fetus. Tissue thromboplastin from the placenta can enter the maternal circulation and cause clotting.
- *Intravascular hemolysis,* where large amounts of free hemoglobin are released into the blood system, incompatible blood transfusions, malaria, and so on.
- *Bacterial and viral infections* that promote platelet aggregation and activation of coagulation system.

DIC is an extremely serious situation, and the laboratory must act quickly to aid the physician in making a proper diagnosis through various coagulation tests. Such tests can include the PT, APTT, coagulation factor assays, FDP testing, platelet count, and so on.

COAGULATION INHIBITORS

A patient may have a bleeding problem associated with acquired circulating anticoagulants directed against a single or several coagulation factors. These can include fibrin-degradation products and malignant paraprotein.

Acquired coagulation inhibitors can be immunoglobulins that are specific antifactor antibodies. The patient has bleeding problems because the factor or factors have been destroyed. In malignant disorders, there may be an interaction between the factor and the inhibitor, forming a complex. However, the factor may be recovered with therapy. Circulating anticoagulants should be strongly suspected when an otherwise healthy individual develops unexplained bleeding or when coagulation tests yield confusing results.

Another anticoagulant that is seen is the lupus anticoagulant. In up to 10% of patients with systemic lupus erythematosus, lupus anticoagulants that can interfere with coagulation are produced.

The APTT test is useful as a screening test for all types of circulating anticoagulants.

HYPERCOAGULABILITY

Hypercoagulability and **thrombosis** are conditions that can be caused by many different situations. Table 8.3 lists several risk factors.

As Table 8.3 illustrates, excessive blood clotting can be caused by many factors, inherited and acquired. Scientists are discovering defects in various aspects of the complex clotting system that can cause blood clots to form. Proteins named *protein C* and *protein S* have been found to play a part in some hypercoagulable states. Congenital deficiencies of these proteins as well as acquired deficiencies (often caused by severe liver disease and acute DIC) can contribute to excessive clotting.

Sensitive assays have been developed to assay the amount of protein C and S present in the body. The PT and the APTT are not sensitive to levels of these proteins. The interested student will further research the antigenic and functional assays developed to test for such proteins.

Table 8.3. Thrombosis Risk Factors

Atherosclerosis
Cigarette use
Hypertension
Diabetes mellitus
LDL cholesterol
Hypertriglyceridemia
Family history
High hemoglobin/hematocrit values
Oral contraceptive use
Obesity
Varicose veins
Infection
Trauma
General anesthesia
Pregnancy
Malignancy
Blood protein defects

SUMMARY

Hemostasis is the mechanism that enables the body to control and stop bleeding from an injured blood vessel. The process is complex and can be visualized as a progression of physical and biological changes.

Coagulation can be divided into primary hemostasis and secondary hemostasis. Primary hemostasis involves the initial changes and responses when an insult to blood vessels occurs. Blood vessels constrict. Platelets secrete chemicals as they stick to the wall of the injured vessel. Secondary hemostasis involves a complex sequence of physiochemical reactions in the body, involving both the intrinsic and extrinsic coagulation systems.

Primary hemostasis testing involves a number of platelet assessments. The most common test for platelets is by automated cell counters. Manual counting techniques include the use of the Unopette® system. The capillary fragility test determines the ability of the capillaries to resist pressure not more than 100 mm Hg. The Ivy bleeding time test using the Simplate® method involves a constant pressure applied above the elbow, using a blood pressure cuff. Bleeding is timed until it ceases. This test is prolonged with very low platelet levels, severe liver disease, and other conditions.

The ability of a normal clot to form is demonstrated by the clot retraction test. A low platelet count or poorly functioning platelets will result in incomplete retraction.

Secondary hemostasis involves stopping the flow of blood in a more stabilized fashion. Coagulation factors are a part of this process, involved in two interrelated systems (the extrinsic and intrinsic pathways) to aid the clotting mechanism. The intrinsic system involves factors I, II, V, VIII, IX, X, XI, and XII, the Fitzgerald factor, and the Fletcher factor. The extrinsic system involves factors I, II, V, VII, and X. All of these factors can be assayed by a variety of manual, semi-automated, and automated techniques, using trisodium citrated blood.

The prothrombin time (PT) is the most commonly ordered test to measure the extrinsic pathway of coagulation. This test is also helpful in monitoring oral anticoagulant therapy. The activated partial thromboplastin time (APTT) is used to detect disorders in the intrinsic clotting system. It can also be used to detect the presence of circulating coagulation inhibitors. Both the PT and the APTT testing is performed on automated instrumentation.

Fibrinolysis is a mechanism in the body that breaks down the clot that has formed to stop bleeding. The fibrinolytic system and the coagulation system are in equilibrium in the normal person to keep the vascular system free of fibrin clots. Tests to assess this system include fibrin-degradation products and D-dimer testing.

Disseminated intravascular coagulation (DIC) is a serious condition in which hemostasis mechanisms are activated, causing intravascular fibrin production and consequent fibrinolysis. DIC can accompany such conditions as obstetrical problems, intravascular hemolysis, and bacterial and viral infections.

Coagulation inhibitors include immunoglobulins that are specific antifactor antibodies and proteins that may be produced in malignant disorders. Patients with lupus can also produce inhibitors.

Hypercoagulability and thrombosis are conditions that can be caused by a variety of conditions, including atherosclerosis, hypertension, oral contraceptive use, pregnancy, malignancy, and other causes. Some of these conditions are inherited, and some are acquired.

REVIEW QUESTIONS

1. When platelets stick together, it is called
   a. adhesion
   b. activation
   c. ecchymoses
   d. platelet aggregation
2. A decreased number of platelets could be recognized by the presence of
   a. petechiae
   b. ecchymoses
   c. gum bleeding
   d. all of the above
3. The prothrombin time (PT) tests which of the following
   a. extrinsic pathway
   b. intrinsic pathway
   c. extrinsic and intrinsic pathways
   d. neither
4. The activated partial thromboplastin time (APTT) tests which of the following
   a. extrinsic pathway
   b. intrinsic pathway
   c. extrinsic and intrinsic pathways
   d. platelet integrity only
5. The coagulation factor associated with hemophilia A is
   a. VIII
   b. VI
   c. XIII
   d. XII
6. In several coagulation procedures, the water bath temperature must be
   a. three degrees below body temperature
   b. three degrees over body temperature
   c. body temperature
   d. you do not employ the use of a water bath in coagulation tests
7. Coagulation testing requires that
   a. the trisodium citrate tube be drawn first
   b. the blood be drawn from the hand
   c. the collection tube must be completely full
   d. the collection tube should be at least half full

8. DIC can be caused by
   a. obstetrical problems
   b. bacterial infections
   c. intravascular hemolysis
   d. all of the above
9. Hypercoagulability means
   a. blood thinning
   b. increased blood clotting
   c. factor VIII deficiency
   d. low platelets

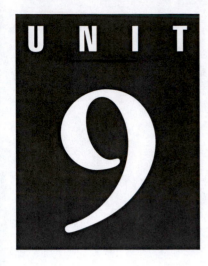

Instrumentation

LEARNING OBJECTIVES

Having completed this unit, it is the responsibility of the student to know the following:

▓ Discuss the two types of automated cell counters commonly used in clinical hematology departments.

▓ Explain the components of a histogram.

▓ Discuss coagulation instrumentation.

▓ Explain the importance of routine instrument maintenance.

GLOSSARY

aperture hole through which cells or particles can pass, being small enough to allow for detection of cells.

electrical impedance interruption in the flow of electricity between two opposite poles.

electrolyte salt solution that allows the flow of electricity through it from a negative to a positive pole.

histogram detailed results obtained from sophisticated cell counters; include graphs of cellular distribution, cell counts, differential determinations, red blood cell indices calculations, and so on.

laser acronym for **l**ight **a**mplified by **s**timulated **e**mission of **r**adiation, referring to an intensified light source.

optical detection counting blood cells by passing a stream of cells through a focused laser beam.

INTRODUCTION

Automation has greatly improved the precision and accuracy of laboratory testing. Many more tests can be run in a normal workday. The more familiar the student is with different systems and with the maintenance of equipment, the more marketable the student is in a job search. Understanding the general principles behind the operation of equipment will help make troubleshooting a problem much easier.

THE CELL COUNTER

There are two means often used to count blood cells and platelets: **electrical impedance** and **optical detection**. Both counting techniques are widely found in the laboratories across the nation. Coulter Electronics (Hialeah, Fla) was the first company to develop cell counting equipment in the 1950s, utilizing the electrical impedance technique. Ortho Diagnostic Systems developed the optical detection technique using **laser** technology.

Both technologies, depending on the sophistication of the equipment, yield a complete blood count including a white and red blood cell count, hemoglobin determination, hematocrit (calculated), red blood cell indices, RDW (red cell distribution width), platelet count, and as much as an eight part differential. Smaller units, found in physicians' offices, may only perform a few of these parameters.

ELECTRICAL IMPEDANCE COUNTING

The electrical impedance counting principle (also called the Coulter principle) is based on diluting a quantity of blood cells in an **electrolyte** (a solution that transmits electricity). The cells are drawn through a small hole called an **aperture**, which has two electrodes placed on either side of the aperture. Electrical potential between the electrodes changes as cells pass. Each time the hole of the aperture is blocked by the cell (or a cell fragment in the case of platelets), the flow of

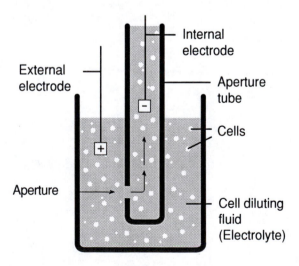

fig. 9.1. Impedance counting (Coulter principle). (From Walters. *Basic Medical Laboratory Techniques.* ed. 5.)

electricity is interrupted. The number of disruptions or pulses is expressed as a particle or cell count. The magnitude of the interruption is correlated with the volume of the particle. Particle size discrimination can be made electronically by setting thresholds above and below which particles will be recognized or ignored. Thousands of particles pass through the aperture in a few seconds, with platelets, white blood cells, and red blood cells being counted simultaneously.

Most cell counters based on electrical impedance have similar construction:

- A *power supply* contains the vacuum and pressure pumps to move liquid through the diluter. This supply also supplies voltages and current needed to sense cells as they pass through openings.
- The *diluter* contains the parts needed to aspirate, pipette, dilute, mix, lyse, and sense the sample. After aspiration, the blood is divided into two parts, each of which is mixed with diluent to form two dilutions. One part goes to the red blood cell aperture bath, where red blood cells and platelets will be counted. The other part goes to the white blood cell bath, where white blood cell information is determined. A lysing reagent is added to the white blood cell bath to lyse the red blood cells and release the hemoglobin. After the white blood cells are counted, the dilution goes into a built-in spectro-photometer to determine the hemoglobin. Rinsing then takes place, and a high vacuum is used to prime the sweep-flow lines and draw off any remaining cells into the vacuum regulator. The aspirator is backwashed to minimize carryover.
- The *analyzer* contains the electronic and computing circuits needed to control the sequence of operations in the diluter and to process the data. The analyzer receives information about size distributions, determining the red cell indices and the red blood cell distribution width (RDW). The analyzer also excludes pulses from cells that did not pass through the center of the openings.

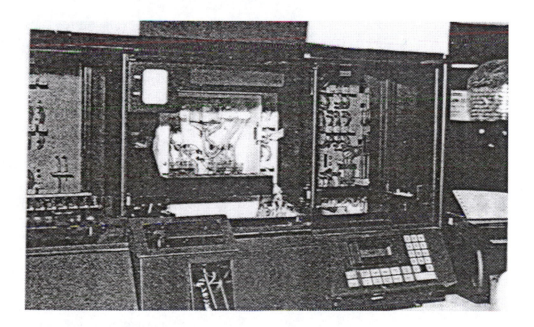

fig. 9.2. Modern cell counter using impedance counting. (From Marshall. *Fundamental Skills for the Clinical Laboratory Professional.* p. 200.)

Many different types of instruments that rely on electrical impedance are available today. Most are sophisticated automated, multiparameter cell counters that can also determine the type of white blood cells present. With this feature, the physician can be given information that is normally contained in a differential. Many laboratories do differential counts only when there are abnormal results in the automated differential performed by the cell counter.

Some sophisticated machines are now designed to have the sampling needle penetrate the stopper of the blood tube, eliminating the need for laboratory professionals to open the blood tube and expose themselves to aerosols, spills, and so on.

OPTICAL DETECTION

The optical detection principle uses laser light to count the cells and size them. As a diluted specimen is passed through a laser beam, each cell interferes with and scatters the light. The amount of light scatter detected by sensors determines the size, density (optical), and number of lobes in the nucleus. The light scattered is detected by another sensor, converting the light to electricity. Each electrical pulse is counted as an individual cell.

These instruments, like the electronic impedance instruments, have an elaborate quality control system for storage of control values, calculations of means, and standard deviations. Levey-Jennings graphs are charted, and flagging of abnormal specimens can be done automatically.

E X E R C I S E  USING THE CELL COUNTER

SAFETY TECHNIQUE: WEAR GLOVES.

Purpose: The cell counting instrument in the hematology laboratory is the most utilized instrument in the department. Understanding the principles of the instrument and proper operation and maintenance is critical for the laboratory professional.

Equipment Needed: Cell counter, EDTA blood sample.

Procedure:
1. If you have a cell counting instrument in the student laboratory, explore the principles involved in the operation of the instrument. If you do not have a counter, this exercise may take the form of a field trip where a laboratory professional will explain the principle of counting cells with a particular instrument. If possible, observe both an electrical impedance counter and an optical detection instrument.
2. Review the start-up procedures for the instrument you are observing.
3. Be able to trace the path of the blood as it travels through the machine. Where are the red blood cells and platelets counted? Where are the white blood cells counted? Which values are calculated?

EXERCISE **85** **USING THE CELL COUNTER** *(continued)*

4. Review quality control measures taken to assure accurate results.
5. Review routine maintenance of the machine to assure proper functioning. Does this machine have a maintenance contract? What maintenance has to be done each day?
6. Go over how the results are delivered. How are abnormal results flagged? What are the procedures for dealing with abnormal results? Which results are considered *panic values?* Is dilution necessary with high counts? How many times are specimens run?
7. If possible, put a specimen of blood through the machine, using proper precautions for handling blood. Run the specimen through again to verify results.

HISTOGRAMS

Modern cell counters do not simply produce blood cell counts. They can also plot graphs showing the cellular size distribution and calculate indices, hematocrits, and RDW determinations. Percentages of types of white blood cells present are also available from some instruments. Results come in the form of **histograms**, a printout produced by some cell counters to give the operator and the physician a detailed patient blood picture.

AUTOMATED DIFFERENTIAL COUNTERS

In the last several years, reliable automated methods for analyzing peripheral blood cell populations have emerged. Automated cell counters are able to provide parameters such as determining percentages of white blood cell populations and identifying samples with abnormalities for further review. Many physicians may want to order a separate differential cell count when abnormalities are suspected. However, the differential results produced by automated cell counters provide good correlations between instrument and manual-derived tests, especially when results are within normal parameters.

Stand-alone automated differential counters are based on the quantitation and evaluation of cell volume, cell light scattering, and cytochemistry, used alone or in combination. Results are expressed in absolute and relative numbers for each cell category.

When results are out of the normal range, some instruments backlight the offending number. Flag indicators can indicate specific locations of abnormalities in the WBC size distribution. The presence of backlighting and/or flagging of results suggests that a manual differential count or careful microscopic scanning of a stained peripheral blood smear is indicated. Health care facility laboratories may set up their own parameters for reviewing abnormal differential slides manually. The manual slide differential may be used when evaluating blood samples from oncology patients and neonatal intensive care populations.

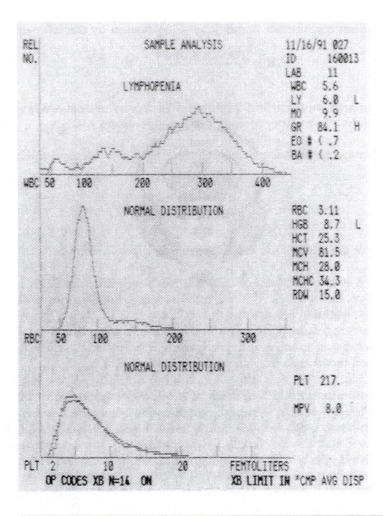

fig. 9.3. Histogram from an automated cell counter. (From Marshall. *Fundamental Skills for the Clinical Laboratory Professional.* p. 353.)

E X E R C I S E　　**86**　　**READING HISTOGRAMS**

Purpose: To become familiar with reading histograms.

Equipment Needed: Normal and abnormal histograms provided by the instructor.

Procedure:
1. Observe and understand the components of the histogram. Make sure you are clear about what each result means.
2. Observe normal patterns of cellular distributions.
3. Notice how abnormal results are flagged on the abnormal examples. How would abnormal results be handled by the operator? When should a physician be called?

EXERCISE **87** **THE AUTOMATED DIFFERENTIAL ANALYSIS**

Purpose: The student observes different methods of automated differential cell counting.

Procedure:

1. At a local clinical laboratory, observe the automated differential values that are generated by both an automated cell counter and a stand-alone differential cell counter.
2. When would laboratory scientists at the facility use the cell counter results? When would an automated differential be ordered? When would a manual cell count be used?
3. Observe the quality control used for each method.

COAGULATION INSTRUMENTATION

Early coagulation instruments tested for the change in optical density of the blood sample as it clotted. These early instruments were not standardized, resulting in inefficiency and lack of precision. Several different types of methods and instruments were developed, including manual methods (see Exercises 88, 89). Today, most manual methods have been replaced by automation. Automated methods include clot elasticity and fibrin adhesion methods, which are used mostly in research, and optical density and electromechanical methods, which are used within the clinical setting.

MECHANICAL CLOT DETECTION

Fibrometers (Figure 9.4) and Dataclot 2 are semiautomated electromechanical machines that measure the flow of electricity and its impedance by the formation of a fibrin clot. In many laboratories this instrument has been used as a backup to the primary coagulation instrument. It consists of three units that are interconnected: the coagulation time unit, the thermal prep block, and the pneumatic pipette.

This instrument can perform several coagulation tests, including the prothrombin time, discussed in Exercise 82.

PHOTO-OPTICAL COAGULATION INSTRUMENTS

The coagulation testing today may be run by fully automated coagulation instrumentation, as seen in Figure 9.5. Some instruments test for a change in optical density, created by clot formation, which is very dense in comparison to the initial solution. These instruments automatically pipette all reagents necessary for testing.

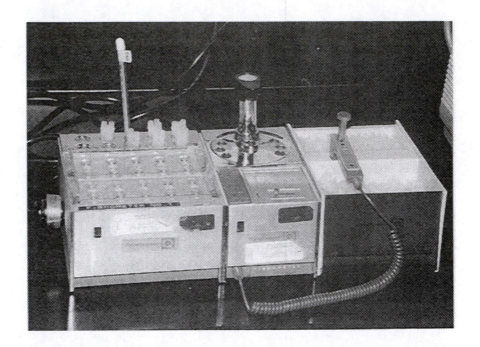

fig. 9.4. Fibrometer. (From Marshall. *Fundamental Skills for the Clinical Laboratory Professional.* p. 459.)

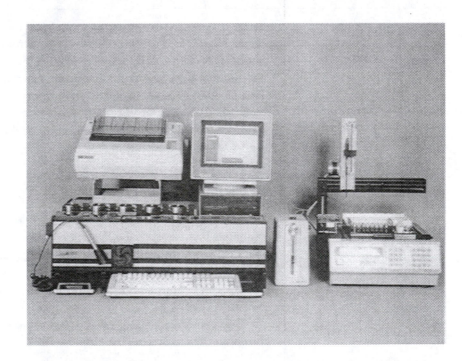

fig. 9.5. Fully automated hemostasis analyzer. (From Marshall. *Fundamental Skills for the Clinical Laboratory Professional.* p. 459.)

EXERCISE **88** **AUTOMATED COAGULATION INSTRUMENTATION**

Purpose: The student is introduced to automated coagulation testing.

Procedure:
1. Visit a clinical laboratory or a coagulation specialty laboratory. Observe various automated coagulation instrumentation.
2. Which are the most common tests run in the laboratory? Which tests are sent to other laboratories, if any?
3. Which tests are most often run STAT?
4. Which tests are ordered when a DIC panel is ordered?
5. Observe all quality control procedures.
6. Ask about preventative maintenance for the various instruments.

PREVENTATIVE MAINTENANCE

All equipment in the hematology laboratory needs to be constantly maintained to function properly. It is the responsibility of every laboratory scientist to participate in this daily activity. Daily records are kept, tracing daily maintenance for each instrument as well as a log of service from outside vendors. Any problems with the instruments are recorded and reported to the laboratory supervisor for appropriate response.

EXERCISE **89** **PERFORMING PREVENTATIVE MAINTENANCE**

SAFETY TECHNIQUE: WEAR GLOVES; BEWARE OF ELECTRICAL WIRES.

Purpose: Preventative maintenance of hematology laboratory instruments is an integral part of a quality control program to assure that accurate results are produced.

Procedure:

Note: If you do not have the machinery in the student laboratory for this exercise, your instructor can request that a laboratory professional in a hematology laboratory go over these procedures with you during a field trip to the facility.

1. Observe external wiring for fraying. Make sure that plugs are properly grounded.

E X E R C I S E **89** **PERFORMING PREVENTATIVE MAINTENANCE**
(continued)

2. Find out where maintenance logs are kept and how they are recorded. Observe troubleshooting logs to see the pattern of problems with the instrument and what was done to solve the problems.
3. Review schedules for cleaning the instrument. If you have a hands-on opportunity, properly clean the instrument.
4. Observe how often controls are run, what types of controls are run, and how they are recorded. Observe control logs (some are kept internally in the machine and results are printed out). If you have a hands-on opportunity, run controls and record results. Do the results fall into proper parameters?
5. Find out about outside maintenance contracts. How frequently is outside maintenance performed? Where are the records kept for outside maintenance?

Preventative maintenance is an integral part of all quality control problems. When hospital inspections are performed, inspectors always carefully go over preventative maintenance logs to assess the quality of work being performed in the laboratory. Poor maintenance can mean compromised results and poor service to patients.

SUMMARY

The use of automated equipment within the hematology laboratory has greatly increased the efficiency of reporting the test results to the physician. It has also increased the accuracy and precision of the laboratory reports.

The most frequently used instrument in the hematology laboratory is the cell counter. Two types of cell counters are currently in popular use—the electrical impedance counter and the optical detection counter. Impedance counting is based on diluting a quantity of blood cells in an electrolyte and drawing the fluid through an aperture. The electrical potential between the electrodes changes as cells pass. Optical detection uses laser light to count the cells and size them.

Modern cell counters do not simply produce blood cell counts; they also plot graphs showing the cellular size distribution. In addition they calculate indices, hematocrits, and RDW distributions. Percentages of white blood cell types are also available; the results of all of these parameters are in the form of histograms.

Automated differential counters include differentials produced by automated cell counters and stand-alone differential counters. Abnormal results are often reviewed by manual differential counts.

Automated coagulation testing is as common now as hematology testing. Some instruments test for a change in optical density, created by clot formation.

Preventative maintenance on all instruments in the hematology laboratory is critical for maintaining a well-functioning quality control program in the laboratory.

REVIEW QUESTIONS

1. When performing a CBC using an automated cell counter, which of the following is important to keep in mind?
   a. that all diluent and lyse fluids are sufficient to complete testing
   b. that all tubing is open to allow free flow of fluids
   c. that all apertures are free of fibrin clots
   d. all of the above
2. The fibrometer
   a. is fully automated
   b. is similiar to a cell counter
   c. relies on optical density
   d. is electromechanical
3. The histogram includes
   a. the white blood cell count
   b. a graphed cell distribution representation
   c. RDW values
   d. all of the above
4. The red cell aperture bath is also the site of counting of
   a. monocytes
   b. platelets
   c. reticulocytes
   d. mononuclear cells
5. Preventative maintenance includes
   a. instrument troubleshooting records
   b. statistics of employees
   c. patient values over several months
   d. patient statistics

UNIT 1 Introduction to Hematology in the Clinical Laboratory

1. b   6. a
2. c   7. b
3. d   8. c
4. c   9. a
5. d   10. b

UNIT 2 Measurement in the Hematology Laboratory

1. b   5. c
2. b   6. c
3. c   7. d
4. a   8. a

UNIT 3 Blood Cell Counting

1. b   6. b
2. a   7. a
3. c   8. a
4. c   9. c
5. b   10. a

UNIT 4 White Blood Cells (Leukocytes)

1. d   9. a
2. b   10. d
3. d   11. c
4. d   12. d
5. c   13. c
6. c   14. c
7. b   15. d
8. b   16. d

UNIT 5 Leukocyte Abnormalities

1. a   9. a
2. b   10. c
3. d   11. d
4. c   12. d
5. d   13. d
6. d   14. d
7. a   15. a
8. d

UNIT 6 Red Blood Cells (Erythrocytes)

1. b	11. d
2. c	12. b
3. b	13. c
4. a	14. d
5. b	15. a
6. d	16. d
7. c	17. c
8. d	18. b
9. b	19. b
10. c	

UNIT 7 Anemias and Hemoglobinopathies

1. c	5. b
2. b	6. b
3. d	7. d
4. b	8. c

UNIT 8 Hemostasis and Coagulation Procedures

1. d	6. c
2. d	7. c
3. a	8. d
4. b	9. b
5. a	

UNIT 9 Instrumentation

1. d	4. b
2. d	5. a
3. d	

REFERENCES

Bennington, James L. *Dictionary and Encyclopedia of Laboratory Medicine and Technology*. Philadelphia: W.B. Saunders Co., 1984.

Brown, Barbara. *Hematology: Principles and Procedures*. Philadelphia: Lea & Febiger, 1993.

Coulter Electronics Corporation. *Instruction and Service Manual*. Hialeah, Fla.

Golde, David W. The Stem Cell. *Scientific American,* December 1991, pp. 86–93.

Harmening, Denise M. *Clinical Hematology and Fundamentals of Hemostasis*. ed. 2. Philadelphia: F.A. Davis Co., 1992.

Howanitz, Joan H. and Peter J. Howanitz. *Laboratory Medicine*. New York: Churchill Livingstone, 1991.

McClatchey, Kenneth D. *Clinical Laboratory Medicine*. Baltimore: Williams and Wilkins, 1994.

McKenzie, Shielyn B. *Textbook of Hematology*. Philadelphia: Lea & Febiger, 1988.

Miale, John B. *Laboratory Medicine Hematology*. ed. 6. St. Louis: The C.V. Mosby Co., 1982.

Pendergraph, Garland E. *Handbook of Phlebotomy*. ed. 2. Philadelphia: Lea & Febiger, 1988.

Powers, Lawrence. *Diagnostic Hematology*. St. Louis: The C.V. Mosby Co., 1989.

Rapaport, Samuel I. *Introduction to Hematology*. ed. 2. Philadelphia: J.B. Lippincott, 1987.

Ravel, Richard. *Clinical Laboratory Medicine*. ed. 2. St. Louis: The C.V. Mosby Co., 1995.

Sheldon, Huntington. *Boyd's Introduction To the Study Of Disease*. ed. 11. Philadelphia: Lea & Febiger, 1992.

Stewart, Charles E. and Koepke, John A. *Basic Quality Assurance Practices for Clinical Laboratories*. New York: Lippincott, 1987.

Tietz, Norbert W. *Clinical Guide to Laboratory Tests*. ed. 3. Philadelphia: W.B. Saunders Co., 1995.

Turgeon, Mary L. *Clinical Hematology: Theory and Procedures*. ed. 2. Boston: Little, Brown and Co., 1993.

Van Wynsberghe, Donna, Noback, Charles R., and Carola, Robert. *Human Anatomy and Physiology*. ed. 3. New York: McGraw-Hill, Inc., 1995.

Wallach, Jacques. *Interpretation of Diagnostic Tests*. ed. 5. Boston: Little, Brown and Company, 1992.

Weisbrot, Irwin M. *Statistics For The Clinical Laboratory*. New York: J.B. Lippincott, 1985.

Williams, M. Ruth and Lindbers, David. *An Introduction To The Profession Of Medical Technology*. ed. 3. Philadelphia: Lea & Febiger, 1979.